ABC OF
ATRIAL FIBRILLATION

ABC OF
ATRIAL FIBRILLATION

edited by

GREGORY Y H LIP MD MRCP DFM FACA

Lecturer in Medicine and Senior Registrar in Cardiology
University Department of Medicine and Department of Cardiology, City Hospital, Birmingham

First published in 1996
by the BMJ Publishing Group, BMA House, Tavistock Square,
London WC1H 9JR

British Library Cataloguing in Publication Data

A catalogue record for this book is available from the
British Library

ISBN 0-7279-1070-1

Typeset by Apek Typesetters Ltd., Nailsea, Bristol
Printed and bound by Craft Print, Singapore

Contents

CONTRIBUTORS

D Gareth Beevers MD FRCP
professor of medicine
University Department of Medicine and Department of Cardiology, City Hospital, Birmingham

John R Coope FRCGP
general practitioner
The Waterhouse, Bollington, near Macclesfield, Derbyshire

Gregory Y H Lip MD MRCP DFM FACA
lecturer in medicine
University Department of Medicine and Department of Cardiology, City Hospital, Birmingham

Gordon D O Lowe MD FRCP
professor of vascular medicine
Haemostasis, Thrombosis and Vascular Medicine Unit, University Department of Medicine, Royal Infirmary, Glasgow

Shyam P Singh MB FRCP
consultant cardiologist
University Department of Medicine and Department of Cardiology, City Hospital, Birmingham

Robert D S Watson MD FRCP
consultant cardiologist
University Department of Medicine and Department of Cardiology, City Hospital, Birmingham

FOREWORD

Most of us have friends or colleagues whose lives are touched or perhaps even devastated by atrial fibrillation. This is no innocuous arrhythmia.

With the advent of radiofrequency ablation, cardiac arrhythmias have garnered new interest and appeal. Atrial fibrillation, however, has remained comparatively neglected. It is the commonest arrhythmia; is is rarely directly fatal yet it creates greater morbidity than probably all the other cardiac arrhythmias put together. Medical therapies directed against atrial fibrillation are modestly effective but all too often their impact is shortlived and the arrhythmia recurs or rate control is lost. This state of affairs was unsatisfactory and clearly could not continue. Not a moment too soon, attention has been turning to atrial fibrillation. Better information regarding its prevalence and the risk factors surrounding its occurrence have been vital for formulating management strategies. Modern critical review of the cost-benefits of treatment options has forced a radical reappraisal of how this arrhythmia should be tackled both in general practice and in the hospital environment. Finally, improved understanding of the mechanism of this complex arrhythmia and a more accurate appreciation of its cellular electrophysiology has prompted the development of new interventional strategies. The field is volatile and exciting but already there are emerging truths that are forming the basis for suggested management strategies. In the course of time they will become the guidelines for dealing with this condition.

The *ABC of Atrial Fibrillation* contains both the old and the new knowledge about this arrhythmia. With each new revelation concerning atrial fibrillation, we must wonder at our predecessors who observed so much and whose writings on this subject are only now being revisited. Decades ago, atrial fibrillation would be defined not just as a single entity but on the basis of the ECG baseline; fine and coarse forms would be identified. These categories were not for mere aesthetic pleasure. Outcome and treatment susceptibility were correlated with different forms. In a much more sophisticated but fundamentally similar way, such details of atrial fibrillation are becoming important again in the 1990s.

There will be new and dramatic developments in atrial fibrillation therapy in the next few years, but for the present this book sets out a logical approach. Facts are presented, management plans are suggested, and the pros and cons of both pharmacological and non-pharmacological therapies are detailed. As beholds modern clinical practice, costs are discussed. Some costs, however, are not detailed as we can only begin to guess at the real community cost of atrial fibrillation.

The *ABC of Atrial Fibrillation* sets out where we now stand and it identifies where the deficiencies lie. There is a great deal of research work ahead before we can feel comfortable that this arrhythmia is under our control. I am certain that the approach of the future will concentrate much more on preventing the disease conditions that create a fibrillatory environment. Aggressive management of disease that is injurious to atrial myocardium will be crucial. Already, such approaches to valvular heart disease are paying dividends and early interventions in myocardial infarction will also likely protect against atrial fibrillation. The management of hypertension and of heart failure should also bring an antiarrhythmic reward in a reduced risk of atrial fibrillation. The *ABC of Atrial Fibrillation* helps us appreciate where these next developments may lie. Its economy, its lack of ambiguity, and its well presented facts are a breath of fresh air in a complex subject area.

Ronald W F Campbell
BHF Professor of Cardiology
Freeman Hospital
University of Newcastle upon Tyne

PREFACE

Atrial fibrillation is the commonest sustained cardiac rhythm disorder. As the elderly population is increasing at twice the rate of the general population and will constitute nearly a quarter of the total population by the turn of the century, atrial fibrillation will become an increasingly common cause of stroke, thromboembolism and heart failure, rendering it as an important new public health problem. Interest in atrial fibrillation has also increased as treatment strategies have improved. For example, atrial fibrillation has long been recognised as a risk factor for stroke, but it is only in the last few years that the efficacy of antithrombotic therapy in prevention against strokes in atrial fibrillation has been well established by prospective clinical studies. The value of atrioventricular node ablation and pacemaker therapy in refractory cases of atrial fibrillation is also increasingly recognised.

Although most doctors, whether in general practice or hospitals, will encounter and have to treat patients with atrial fibrillation, there continues to be confusion and considerable variation in management strategies, especially between cardiologists and non-cardiologists. Guidelines on the management of this common disorder are therefore required. The *ABC of Atrial Fibrillation* reviews the epidemiology, pathophysiology, clinical features, and differential diagnosis of atrial fibrillation; and suggests a logical strategy for the managment of such patients. The use of non-pharmaceutical approaches and drugs (including antiarrhythmic and antithrombotic therapy) are discussed, and the relevance of atrial fibrillation to general practice and hospital practice are reviewed. It is sincerely hoped that this concise book will bring order and greater understanding to the management of atrial fibrillation, where confusion and chaos were previously evident.

Gregory Y H Lip

1 HISTORY, EPIDEMIOLOGY, AND IMPORTANCE OF ATRIAL FIBRILLATION

Gregory Y H Lip, D Gareth Beevers

> "When the pulse is irregular and tremulous and the beats occur at intervals, then the impulse of life fades; when the pulse is slender (smaller than feeble, but still perceptible, thin like a silk thread), then the impulse of life is small."
>
> Huang Ti Nei Ching Su Wên

Presenting symptoms in emergency admissions with atrial fibrillation

Dyspnoea—52%
Chest pain—34%
Palpitation—26%
Dizziness or syncope—19%

Atrial fibrillation is the commonest sustained disorder of cardiac rhythm. When it is present many prognostic and therapeutic implications exist as overall morbidity and mortality increase appreciably. Despite this, atrial fibrillation is sometimes regarded as a fairly trivial and unimportant disorder and is often neglected, probably because many patients have few symptoms. In fact, some patients with chronic atrial fibrillation may require long term treatment with potent antiarrhythmic and anticoagulant drugs, which may have important pharmacological interactions and adverse effects. In addition, treatment differs importantly for chronic and paroxysmal atrial fibrillation and for atrial fibrillation, atrial flutter, and the other supraventricular arrhythmias.

Atrial fibrillation is encountered in many clinical settings. It may, for example, be discovered incidentally in an asymptomatic patient, develop in a patient who merely has a chest infection, or be found in a patient with a ventricular rate of 200 beats/min who is too lightheaded to stand up. Patients admitted with atrial fibrillation may have many cardiorespiratory symptoms and clinical features, including syncope and stroke.

A brief history

History of atrial fibrillation

Adams, 1827
Probably the first to recognise the condition clinically but as a "sign of mitral stenosis"
Bouillaud, 1835
Found that digitalis reduced the ventricular rate dramatically even though irregularity of pulse persisted
Hope, 1839
Identified irregular pulse in association with mitral stenosis—exercise worsened the total irregularity, whereas it abolished an intermittent pulse
Marey, 1863
Published a pulse tracing of atrial fibrillation from a patient with mitral stenosis
Roberts, 1873
Found that digitalis relieved the pulmonary symptoms of mitral disease especially in the presence of irregularity of the heart
Vulpian, 1874
Observed atrial fibrillation in vivo (dog)
Engelmann, 1894
Reported atrial fibrillation caused by multiple foci in the atria
Einthoven, 1900
Invented the electrocardiograph
Lewis, 1909
Recorded atrial fibrillation with electrocardiograph; studied mechanisms of the condition
Rothberger and Winterberg, 1909
Identified "arrhythmia perpetua" and "fibrillation of the auricles"
Lown, 1969
Recommended cardioversion of atrial fibrillation

Perhaps the earliest description of atrial fibrillation is in *The Yellow Emperor's Classic of Internal Medicine* (Huang Ti Nei Ching Su Wên). The legendary emperor physician is believed to have ruled China between 1696 and 2598 BC. The poor prognosis associated with chaotic irregularity of the pulse was clearly acknowledged by most of the ancient physicians, but in recorded history, William Harvey in 1628 was probably the first to describe "fibrillation of the auricles" in animals.

In clinical practice and with the aid of Laénnec's recently invented stethoscope, Robert Adams reported in 1827, the association of irregular pulses with mitral stenosis; in 1863, Etienne Marey published a pulse tracing from such a patient. Other early descriptions of atrial fibrillation and its importance were published early this century by Sir James Mackenzie and Heinrich Hering.

The discovery of the therapeutic properties of digitalis leaf (*Digitalis purpurea*) in 1785 by William Withering brought some relief to patients with severe heart failure. It is interesting that Withering recorded a patient who had a weak, irregular pulse that became "more full and more regular" after five draughts containing *Fol Digital Purp oz iv*. In 1835 Jean Baptiste Bouillaud said that he considered digitalis to be "a sort of opium for the heart."

History, epidemiology, and importance of atrial fibrillation

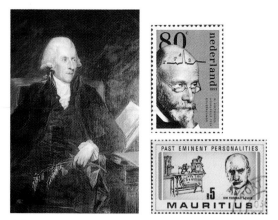

Left: William Withering. Right: (top) Willem Einthoven; (bottom) Thomas Lewis.

The main diagnostic breakthrough was the invention of the electrocardiograph by Willem Einthoven in 1900. A close friend of Einthoven, Sir Thomas Lewis at University College Hospital, London, was the first to record an electrocardiogram in a patient with atrial fibrillation.

The exact mechanisms and importance of atrial fibrillation remained controversial (Lewis and Mackenzie had disagreed about these issues) until 1970, when Bootsma and co-workers, with the aid of computers, concluded that the totally irregular response of the ventricles was due to the effect of "randomly spaced atrial impulses of random strength reaching the atrioventricular node from random directions."

The epidemiological importance of atrial fibrillation as an important precursor of cardiac and cerebrovascular death was investigated in detail in the Framingham study by William Kannell and colleagues in 1982. Over the past 10 years, awareness has increased of the hazards of sustained non-rheumatic atrial fibrillation and the benefits of prophylaxis against thrombosis in preventing cerebral thromboembolism.

Epidemiology

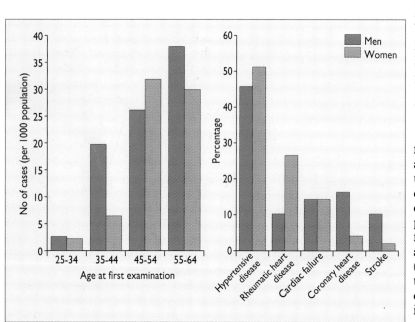

Left: Cumulative incidence of atrial fibrillation over 22 years. Right: Previous cardiovascular disease in patients with atrial fibrillation.

Atrial fibrillation is common in the community, affecting up to 5% of people aged 75 or over. It is a major reason for emergency admissions and cause of cardiovascular deaths. Thus most clinicians in hospital and general practice will participate in managing such patients. As the prevalence of the condition increases with age, atrial fibrillation will become increasingly common in the increasingly aging population.

Estimates of the prevalence of atrial fibrillation in the community vary widely around the world. To date, British studies of the prevalence of atrial fibrillation in the community have involved small numbers of elderly patients from unrepresentative populations. There have been recent appeals for further information on the prevalence of atrial fibrillation in Britain, the prevalence of (and contraindications to) anticoagulant treatment, and the factors that influence doctors' decisions in treating atrial fibrillation, including the investigation of patients with this arrhythmia. An understanding of these factors is required for health care provision, especially with regard to the optimum methods of investigation of patients and a greater appreciation of the role of antithrombotic therapy.

Epidemiological studies have shown that atrial fibrillation is fairly uncommon in people aged under 50 years but is found in 0·5% of people aged 50–59, increasing to 8·8% at age 80–89. Furthermore, the arrhythmia may be either chronic or paroxysmal. In the Framingham study, hypertension, cardiac failure, and rheumatic heart disease were the commonest precursors of atrial fibrillation. Up to a third of patients with atrial fibrillation, however, may have idiopathic or "lone" atrial fibrillation, where no precipitating cause can be identified and no evidence of structural heart disease exists.

Atrial fibrillation is more common in hospital practice than in general practice, being present in up to 7% of emergency medical admissions to district general hospitals. The commonest causes in Western countries

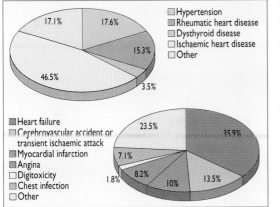

Hypertension
Rheumatic heart disease
Dysthyroid disease
Ischaemic heart disease
Other

17.1% 17.6% 15.3% 46.5% 3.5%

Heart failure
Cerebrovascular accident or transient ischaemic attack
Myocardial infarction
Angina
Digitoxicity
Chest infection
Other

23.5% 35.9% 7.1% 1.8% 8.2% 10% 13.5%

Top: Causes of atrial fibrillation among emergency admissions to hospital. Bottom: Presenting clinical features on admission.

include coronary heart disease, hypertension, and rheumatic and non-rheumatic valve heart disease. The commonest presenting features included heart failure, stroke, chest pain (including myocardial infarction or angina), and respiratory diseases. By contrast, in developing countries rheumatic heart disease is by far the commonest cause of atrial fibrillation.

In general practice, while atrial fibrillation is the commonest cardiac arrhythmia, in many patients the condition remains unrecognised. In a screening programme in patients aged 65–74; 3·4% were found to have atrial fibrillation (J R Coope, unpublished observations). A strong case for long term anticoagulation could be made in up to 80% of these patients. In a single general practice population in Tamworth, screening a total of 819 patients aged over 65 years found 30 patients who were in atrial fibrillation (3·7%) (Hill et al 1987). In a study from a general practice in Sussex, only 106 patients were studied from a total of 268 patients aged 75 years or over, with atrial fibrillation being documented in 8 patients (Camm et al 1980). The feasibility of diagnosing and managing these patients presents a clinical challenge for primary health care teams.

Importance

> All doctors and hospital and primary care nurses must be trained to detect and manage atrial fibrillation

Importance of treating atrial fibrillation

To relieve symptoms of congestive heart failure, hypotension, or angina that can be directly attributed to a rapid heart rate

To improve overall cardiac function

To improve exercise tolerance

To reduce the risk of thromboembolism and stroke

Summary

Atrial fibrillation
- Common arrhythmia with different causes, clinical presentations, and treatment options
- Wide variations in management strategies
- Three phases of management are essential:
  Search for underlying cause
  Control arrhythmia and reduce thromboembolic risk
  Consider cardioversion to sinus rhythm if appropriate

Because of the serious implications of atrial fibrillation, clinicians in all specialties, as well as hospital and primary health care nurses, must be adequately trained in its detection and management. The sudden onset of fast atrial fibrillation may precipitate overt heart failure, particularly if left ventricular function is already compromised by coexisting heart disease, such as valve or ischaemic heart disease. Less dramatic presentations of atrial fibrillation include palpitations, dyspnoea, angina, and general fatigue or lethargy. Symptoms may be more pronounced on exercise, with a greatly limited exercise tolerance.

More important, however, is the finding that non-rheumatic atrial fibrillation increases the risk of stroke by a factor of five. The risk of stroke in someone with atrial fibrillation is about 5% a year, and epidemiological evidence suggests that this risk increases with age, blood pressure, and other evidence of heart disease. Atrial fibrillation may also increase the risk of recurrent stroke. Patients with acute stroke and atrial fibrillation have a significantly higher mortality than patients in sinus rhythm.

Therapeutic benefits from treating atrial fibrillation have been proved. The main priorities are to ameliorate the adverse haemodynamic effects of the poor cardiac output related to the arrhythmia and to reduce thromboembolic risks of atrial fibrillation. Electrical and pharmacological cardioversion to, and the maintenance of, normal sinus rhythm remains the optimal strategy to enhance cardiac performance and reduce the thromboembolic risk. As cardiac function and exercise tolerance may improve after cardioversion, cardioversion should be increasingly considered. The use of this option, however, varies among clinicians and among medical centres, as does the use of anticoagulants before and after cardioversion.

Key references

Camm JC, Evans KE, Ward DE, Martin A. The rhythm of the heart in active elderly subjects. *Am Heart J* 1980;**99**:598–603.

Flegel KM. From delirium cordis to atrial fibrillation: historical development of a disease concept. *Ann Intern Med* 1995;**122**:867–73.

Hill JD, Mottram EM, Killeen PD. Study of the prevalence of atrial fibrillation in general practice patients over 65 years of age. *J R Coll Gen Pract* 1987;**37**:172–3.

Kannel WB, Abbott RD, Savage DD, McNamara PM. Epidemiological features of chronic atrial fibrillation. The Framingham study. *N Engl J Med* 1982;**306**:1018–22.

Lown B. Electrical reversion of cardiac arrhythmias. *Br Heart J* 1967;**29**:469–89.

Lip GYH, Tean KN, Dunn FG. Treatment of atrial fibrillation in a district general hospital. *Br Heart J* 1994;**71**:92–5.

Krikler DM. The Foxglove, "The old woman from Shropshire", and William Withering. *J Am Coll Cardiol* 1985;**5**:3A–9A.

The role of anticoagulant drugs as prophylaxis against thromboembolism in patients with atrial fibrillation has attracted much interest recently. The results of several recent, large, prospective randomised controlled trials consistently show that anticoagulation reduces the risk of strokes by about two thirds without a significant excess of adverse effects. These studies have therefore established the role of oral anticoagulant drugs in atrial fibrillation. Physicians continue to be reluctant, however, to introduce this treatment, with an appreciable proportion of patients still not being given anticoagulant drugs despite an absence of contraindications.

The sources of the data presented in the illustrations are: Kannel *et al*, *N Engl J Med* 1982;**306**:1018-22 for the graphs of incidence of atrial fibrillation and previous cardiovascular disease; and Lip *et al*, *Br Heart J* 1994;**71**:92-5 for the pie charts of causes of atrial fibrillation among emergency admissions to hospital and presenting clinical features on admission. The source of the information in the box on the history of fibrillation is Acierno LJ. *The history of cardiology*. New York: Parthenon Publishing, 1994. The painting of William Withering is reproduced with permission of the University of Birmingham.

2 AETIOLOGY, PATHOPHYSIOLOGY, AND CLINICAL FEATURES

Gregory Y H Lip, D Gareth Beevers, Shyam P Singh, Robert D S Watson

Aetiology

Causes of atrial fibrillation

Cardiac causes	Non-cardiac causes
Common	
Ischaemic heart disease	Thyrotoxicosis
Hypertension	Acute infections, especially pneumonia
Rheumatic heart disease	Excess alcohol intake
Sick sinus syndrome	Lung carcinoma
Pre-excitation syndromes (for example, Wolff-Parkinson-White)	Other intrathoracic pathology (for example, pleural effusion)
	Postoperative problems, especially after thoracotomy or coronary artery bypsss
Less common	
Cardiomyopathy or heart muscle disease	Pulmonary thromboemolism
Pericardial disease, including effusion and constrictive pericarditis	
Atrial septal defect	
Atrial myxoma	

> **Left ventricular hypertrophy is considered to be present if the left ventricular mass index is > 134 g/m² in men and > 110 g/m² in women**

Ischaemic heart disease

Ischaemic heart disease is probably the most common underlying cause of atrial fibrillation in Britain. However, much depends on the criteria used for diagnosis. Many epidemiological studies have depended on electrocardiogram criteria or clinical history. Indeed, studies depending on ST-T wave abnormalities only on the electrocardiogram may encounter difficulties in interpretation, especially if the patient is taking digoxin or has left ventricular hypertrophy. The frequency of coronary disease (or other aetiological causes) also depends on the type of study population.

In hospital based populations ischaemic heart disease was the commonest aetiological factor, followed by hypertension and valve disease. By contrast, population studies such as the Framingham and the Manitoba follow upstudies reported that hypertension was the most common aetiological factor.

Unfortunately, there have been few population based studies in Britain, and published studies have been criticised as being performed in unrepresentative populations.

In addition, the fast ventricular rate due to atrial fibrillation may cause angina, leading to cardiac ischaemia and heart failure. Atrial fibrillation may complicate acute myocardial infarction in 10–15% of cases and is often a marker of extensive, myocardial damage and a poor prognosis, with increased mortality. If atrial fibrillation occurs with an acute myocardial infarction, it tends to occur in the first 24 hours and is usually self limiting. Patients should be observed unless fast atrial fibrillation occurs or the patient is haemodynamically compromised; in the event of the latter, urgent DC cardioversion may be necessary.

Atrial fibrillation is also a marker of underlying ventricular dysfunction and a compromised myocardium. Many years after myocardial infarction, ventricular scarring and dilatation often predispose to atrial fibrillation and congestive heart failure.

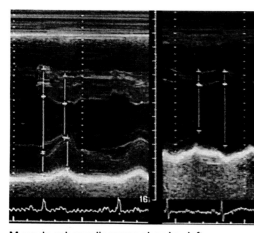

M mode echocardiograms showing left ventricular hypertrophy (left) and normal heart (right).

Hypertension

Hypertension accounted for about half of the cases of atrial fibrillation in the Framingham study. Hypertension contributes to the complications of stroke and thromboembolism in such patients, especially if left ventricular hypertrophy is present. Electrocardiography is useful for screening for left ventricular hypertrophy (for example, with the criteria of Sokolow and Lyon—S wave in V1 and R wave in V5 or V6 of ≥ 35 mm), and if the electrocardiogram is abnormal the echocardiogram will invariably show left ventricular hypertrophy. Left ventricular

Aetiology, pathophysiology, and clinical features

hypertrophy on echocardiography is defined by calculating the left ventricular mass index.

Atrial fibrillation may be secondary to left atrial dilatation, which occurs in hypertensive patients, as a consequence of reduced left ventricular compliance. In addition, hypertension may be associated with underlying coronary artery disease, which itself is a risk for atrial fibrillation and thromboembolism.

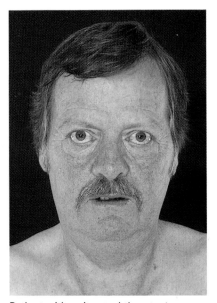

Patient with goitre and thyrotoxic eye disease (published with patient's permission).

Rheumatic heart disease

In a survey of emergency admissions of patients with atrial fibrillation, rheumatic heart disease (predominantly mitral valve disease) was present in 15% of cases. Rheumatic valve disease, especially mitral valve stenosis, is particularly important as it increases the thromboembolic risk of patients with chronic atrial fibrillation about 18-fold. Up to a fifth of patients with mitral stenosis and atrial fibrillation develop embolic events, which in most (60–75%) cases affect the cerebral circulation. This risk of stroke and thromboembolism for patients in atrial fibrillation is three to seven times that of patients with mitral stenosis in sinus rhythm. Echocardiography in such cases may show left atrial thrombus, although transthoracic echocardiography is not a sensitive or reliable method of detection. Transoesophageal echocardiography is an important advance in imaging left atrial thrombus.

Thyroid disease

Thyrotoxicosis is an important and curable cause of atrial fibrillation. About 10–15% of patients with untreated thyrotoxicosis develop atrial fibrillation. Thyrotoxicosis may be underdiagnosed, however, as thyroid function tests are often neglected, particularly in elderly people, in whom classic signs of thyrotoxicosis may not be obvious. One clinical clue may be the failure of digoxin to control the ventricular rate without the addition of β blockers. Hyperthyroidism (affecting about 1% of the population) may also coexist with both ischaemic and rheumatic heart disease. Thyroid function tests should therefore be routinely checked in atrial fibrillation of recent onset.

Rarely, hypothyroidism may cause heart muscle disease and heart failure. Myxoedema is also associated with hyperlipidaemia and an increased risk of heart disease.

Excess alcohol intake

Atrial fibrillation due to an excess intake of alcohol often occurs after holidays or at weekends, giving rise to the term "holiday heart syndrome." Alcohol can thus precipitate atrial fibrillation in healthy people (with otherwise normal hearts), who may have no subsequent risk of atrial fibrillation. Chronic excess intake of alcohol can also be associated with a dilated heart (alcoholic heart muscle disease) and atrial fibrillation.

Pneumonia

Pneumonia is commonly associated with atrial fibrillation in medical patients admitted urgently, being present in about 7% of cases. It is often difficult to know, however, whether the pneumonia is complicating pre-existing atrial fibrillation or is the precipitant of atrial fibrillation. Pneumonia as a precipitant of atrial fibrillation occurs predominantly in elderly patients, who thus have an acute precipitating cause for atrial fibrillation. The pneumonia should therefore be treated and cardioversion to sinus rhythm after treatment of the acute episode should be considered.

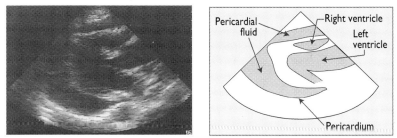

Two dimensional echocardiogram (and diagram) showing large pericardial effusion

Other causes

Other cardiac causes of atrial fibrillation include congenital heart disease (especially atrial septal defect), the sick sinus syndrome, and the pre-excitation syndromes associated with accessory pathways in the conducting system of the heart (such as the Wolff-Parkinson-White syndrome). Idiopathic dilated and hypertrophic cardiomyopathy and pericardial diseases (such as pericardial effusion) are also associated with atrial fibrillation.

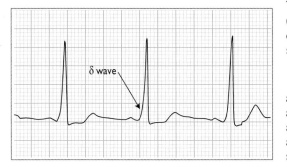

Electrocardiogram showing short PR interval and δ wave in Wolff-Parkinson-White syndrome.

An atrial septal defect should be considered in a young patient with atrial fibrillation, especially if a pulmonary ejection systolic murmur in association with a split, second heart sound is heard. The Wolff-Parkinson-White syndrome is recognised by a short PR interval (<0.12 seconds in an electrocardiogram) and a δ wave in the electrocardiogram when the patient is in sinus rhythm, and should be suspected in a young patient presenting with fast atrial fibrillation.

Non-cardiac causes of atrial fibrillation are also often encountered, and causes of single, isolated episodes include pneumonia (and other acute infections); lung tumours and other intrathoracic conditions, such as pleural effusions; pulmonary thromboembolism; and surgery. When atrial fibrillation occurs postoperatively, it is usually after cardiothoracic surgery, although any surgery with general anaesthesia may precipitate atrial fibrillation. The incidence of supraventricular arrhythmias after cardiothoracic surgery is 20%. Atrial fibrillation after cardiothoracic surgery often requires treatment in the short term. In contrast, atrial fibrillation after non-cardiothoracic surgery is usually self limiting, often reverting spontaneously to sinus rhythm.

Features of "idiopathic" or "lone" atrial fibrillation

Diagnosis of exclusion
No history of cardiovascular disease or hypertension
No abnormal cardiac signs on physical examination
Normal chest x ray film and electrocardiogram (apart from the atrial fibrillation) with no previous myocardial infarction or left ventricular hypertrophy
Normal atria, valves, and left ventricular size (and function) on echocardiography

---

Idiopathic or "lone" atrial fibrillation

Some patients with atrial fibrillation have no predisposing factor or cardiac lesions. The condition in these patients is classified as "lone" or "idiopathic" atrial fibrillation. Lone atrial fibrillation can be either paroxysmal or persistent, and is present in between 3% and 11% of all patients with atrial fibrillation.

Young patients (aged under 60 years) with lone atrial fibrillation are generally accepted to be at a low thromboembolic risk, and antithrombotic treatment may not be justified. Data from the Framingham study, however, suggest a fivefold increase in the incidence of stroke in elderly patients (aged over 65) with the condition, and antithrombotic treatment should be considered.

Pathophysiology and electrophysiology

Haemodynamic disturbances

Fast ventricular rate
Reduced diastolic filling period, especially with sudden changes to a very rapid heart rate, results in a further reduction in cardiac output (especially with valvar stenosis or reduced left ventricular compliance— for example, in left ventricular hypertrophy)
Reduced atrial transport (lack of organised atrial mechanical activity with a concomitant decrease in stroke volume and cardiac output)
Atrial dilatation and loss of atrial systole, leading to intra-atrial stasis, which favours formation of thrombi
Onset of a rapid ventricular response may also lead to some mitral incompetence, thus further reducing forward flow

---

The haemodynamic disturbance of atrial fibrillation results essentially from the absence of atrial systole ("atrial kick") and from the rapidity and irregularity of the ventricular response, with a consequent loss of cardiac output (a loss of about 10% in normal individuals, with a greater loss at fast ventricular rates). This is more important in patients with increasing age or with progressive impairment of left ventricular contraction, or with both, in whom atrial systole contributes increasingly towards the overall stroke volume.

Aetiology, pathophysiology, and clinical features

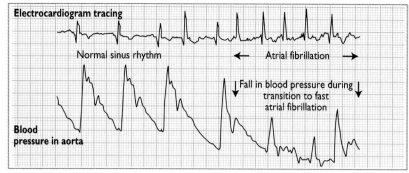

Blood pressure trace showing fall in blood pressure after onset of fast atrial fibrillation.

A rapid heart rate reduces the diastolic filling interval, and the additional loss of the sequential atrioventricular contraction mechanism in atrial fibrillation may lead to a dramatic reduction in cardiac output and to other haemodynamic disturbances. This is substantiated by evidence of a much improved cardiac output after cardioversion of atrial fibrillation to sinus rhythm.

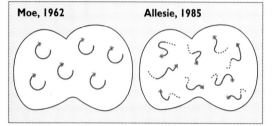

Electrophysiology of atrial fibrillation: Moe's model, multiple coexisting re-entrant wavefronts of activation within atria; and Allesie's model, multiple wavelets continually sweeping around atria in irregular, shifting patterns.

The electrophysiological mechanism of atrial fibrillation is thought to involve several coexisting re-entrant wavefronts continuously sweeping around the atria, repeatedly encountering excitable myocardium. Several factors predispose to long term maintenance of the arrhythmia: atrial enlargement (for example, secondary to mitral valve disease, hypertension), fibrosis of atrial tissue (resulting in slowing of intra-atrial conduction), and altered autonomic tone, especially increased sympathetic activity. In addition, heterogeneity of atrial refractoriness and slow conduction times (allowing time for the myocardium to regain excitability between each wavefront) help to perpetuate the process, leading to long term atrial fibrillation.

Clinical features

Symptoms with atrial fibrillation

Often none
Limited exercise tolerance (dyspnoea, fatigue)
Angina
Palpitation
Presyncope and syncope
Heart failure
Stroke

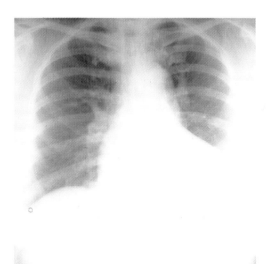

Chest radiograph showing cardiomegaly and pulmonary oedema.

Atrial fibrillation commonly presents as reduced exercise tolerance and heart failure. Less dramatic presentations include dyspnoea, angina, palpitation, and dizziness. Syncope is rare with atrial fibrillation, unless associated with the sick sinus syndrome or pre-excitation syndromes, such as the Wolff-Parkinson-White syndrome. The symptoms may be more pronounced on exercise, as a rapid ventricular response may substantially impair exercise tolerance. Occasionally patients may present as an emergency with a combination of presyncope, syncope, fatigue, dyspnoea, and lethargy, and quite commonly with gross pulmonary oedema, angina, cerebral underperfusion, and stroke. Physical findings include a pulse that is irregular in rate, rhythm, and volume; variable intensity of the first heart sound; and absence of "a" waves in the jugular venous pulse, resulting in a single positive waveform being discerned. With fast ventricular rates, an apex-radial pulse deficit appears, as each contraction may not be sufficiently strong to transmit an arterial pulse wave through the peripheral artery. Measurement of ventricular rates (at rest and on exercise) may be useful in assessing the efficacy of drug treatment in atrial fibrillation.

Heart failure

The sudden onset of fast atrial fibrillation may often precipitate overt heart failure, particularly if left ventricular function is already compromised by coexisting heart disease—for example, valvar or ischaemic heart disease. Heart failure is associated with atrial fibrillation in about 35% of cases. In these patients, atrial fibrillation may be a marker of increased mortality and may also enhance the substantial risk of thromboembolism.

Stroke

Non-rheumatic atrial fibrillation increases fivefold the risk of stroke and is present in about 15% of patients presenting with acute stroke. The risk of stroke in someone with atrial fibrillation is about 5% a year, and epidemiological evidence suggests that this risk increases with age, raised blood pressure, and other evidence of heart disease.

Key reference

Murgatroyd FD, Camm AJ. Atrial arrhythmias. *Lancet* 1993;**341**:1317–22.

Patients with atrial fibrillation may also have an increased risk of recurrent stroke and have silent cerebral infarcts (often multiple) on computed tomography. In addition, patients with acute stroke and atrial fibrillation have a significantly higher mortality than patients in sinus rhythm (23% v 8% in the Oxfordshire Community Stroke Project). This higher mortality is explained partly by the association of atrial fibrillation with large, total anterior cerebral infarcts, probably due to occlusion of the middle cerebral artery.

Thromboembolism

Atrial fibrillation predisposes to the formulation of intracardiac thrombus, which may result in stroke and thromboembolism. The commonest site of thrombus is the left atrial appendage. Right atrial thrombus with subsequent pulmonary thromboembolism is a rare complication.

3 DIFFERENTIAL DIAGNOSIS OF ATRIAL FIBRILLATION

Gregory Y H Lip, Robert D S Watson

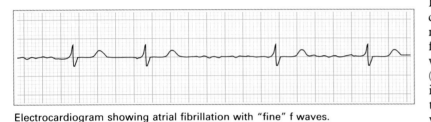

Electrocardiogram showing atrial fibrillation with "fine" f waves.

During atrial fibrillation the atrial impulses discharge at a rate of 350–600 per minute, resulting in small (or "fine"), irregular f (fibrillation) waves. The amplitude of these waves varies and may be especially prominent (or "coarse") in lead V1. As only occasional impulses penetrate the atrioventricular node, a totally irregular ventricular rhythm results, which is the characteristic of this arrhythmia.

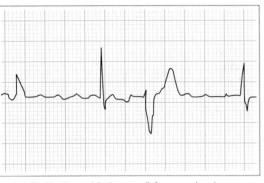

Atrial fibrillation with "coarse" f waves (and ventricular ectopic).

Rapid atrial fibrillation with a rapid ventricular response may easily be mistaken for other supraventricular arrhythmias—for example, atrial flutter or supraventricular tachycardias. Variation in the RR interval is the important clue. At very high heart rates, with a short RR interval, beat to beat variation may be subtle but may become more obvious if the carotid sinus is massaged or the speed of the electrocardiogram trace increased. In a young patient with fast atrial fibrillation it is important to consider an underlying pre-excitation syndrome, such as the Wolff-Parkinson-White syndrome, as traditional drugs such as digoxin or verapamil will accelerate the ventricular response by blocking atrioventricular node impulses and increasing conduction through the accessory pathway.

Finally, atrial fibrillation with a bundle branch block pattern on the QRS complex may be difficult to distinguish from a ventricular tachycardia: again, the important difference is the irregularity of the RR interval present in atrial fibrillation.

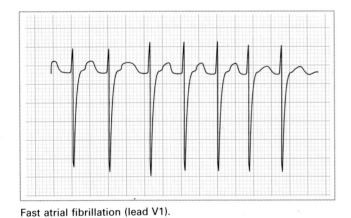

Fast atrial fibrillation (lead V1).

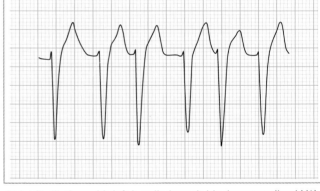

Atrial fibrillation with left bundle branch block pattern (lead V1).

Atrial extrasystoles

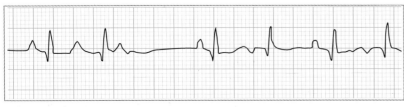

Sinus rhythm with multiple atrial extrasystoles. Note varying morphology of P waves and that P waves may be difficult to discern (for example, "hidden" in T wave of first complex).

Atrial extrasystoles occur commonly and may account for an irregular pulse, leading to atrial fibrillation being wrongly diagnosed. Long pauses may follow as sinus node automaticity is depressed by the extrasystole. multifocal extrasystoles are particularly common in pulmonary disease.

Sinus tachycardia

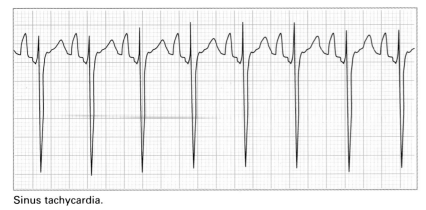

Sinus tachycardia.

Sinus tachycardia is a sinus rhythm of over 100 beats/min. A sinus tachycardia has a gradual onset and offset. P waves (most easily seen in leads II or V1) precede each QRS complex; at very fast heart rates these waves may be difficult to discern, and the rhythm may be confused with fast atrial fibrillation. Distinction from atrial fibrillation thus depends on awareness of the irregular ventricular rate of atrial fibrillation. In cases of apparent sinus tachycardia at rest it is also important to exclude atrial tachycardia or atrial flutter.

Supraventricular arrhythmias

Supraventricular arrhythmias

Atrial fibrillation

Atrial flutter

Supraventricular tachycardias
- Atrial tachycardias
- Junctional tachycardias
  Atrioventricular nodal re-entry tachycardias, with a micro re-entry circuit in the atrioventricular node
  Atrioventricular re-entry tachycardias, with bypass tract present—for example, the Wolff-Parkinson-White and Lown-Ganong-Levine syndromes

A simplified classification of supraventricular arrhythmias is shown in the box. Apart from atrial fibrillation and atrial flutter (which are usually classified and managed differently), other supraventricular arrhythmias are commonly regarded as supraventricular tachycardias. The arrhythmia commonly referred to as a paroxysmal supraventricular tachycardia in clinical practice usually refers to an atrioventricular re-entrant tachycardia.

Atrial flutter

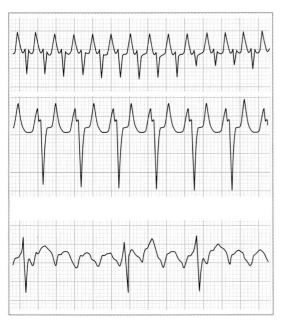

Top: Atrial flutter with 1:1 conduction. Centre: Same patient with atrial flutter and 2:1 block after intravenous adenosine. Bottom: Atrial flutter with variable block.

In atrial flutter there is a re-entrant circuit within the atria, resulting in the atria discharging at about 300 beats/min. Most commonly, the circuit lies within the right atrium and is conducted along the lateral right atrium and "returns" superiorly along the atrial septum.

Atrial discharges result in the characteristic F (flutter) waves—resulting in a sawtoothed pattern—which are best seen in leads II, III and aVF or in V1. The conducting ability of the atrioventricular node determines the ventricular response. Most commonly, alternate atrial implulses are conducted to the ventricles, resulting in a ventricular rate close to 150 beats/min—that is, atrial flutter with 2:1 block. Certain drugs, such as digoxin, adenosine, or verapamil or impaired atrioventricular conduction may lead to more atrioventricular block—for example, 3:1 or 4:1. Atrial flutter with variable atrioventricular block is commonly confused with atrial fibrillation.

The use of class I agents, such as quinidine or disopyramide, in patients with atrial flutter may accelerate the ventricular response with a 1:1 atrioventricular conduction. This may be due in part to the atrial rate slowing and the anticholinergic effects (especially with quinidine and disopyramide), which result in an increase in atrioventricular conduction. With atrial flutter class 1 agents should therefore be given with digoxin, β blockers, or verapamil to avoid possible accelerated atrioventricular conduction.

Differential diagnosis of atrial fibrillation

Atrial flutter may sometimes degenerate into atrial fibrillation, which is easier to treat pharmacologically than atrial flutter. Commonly used drugs that act at the atrioventricular node, such as digoxin, occasionally convert atrial flutter to atrial fibrillation.

Atrial tachycardia

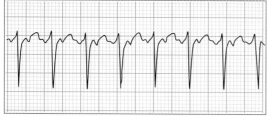

Atrial tachycardia.

Atrial tachycardia is commonly confused with atrial flutter or fast atrial fibrillation. The main difference is that the atrial rate in atrial tachycardia is slower, at 120–250 beats/min. Atrioventricular block (which may be variable) may coexist. This arrhythmia accounts for only around 10% of supraventricular tachycardias. Paroxysmal atrial tachycardia with block is commonly associated with digoxin toxicity, which may have been given originally to control atrial fibrillation.

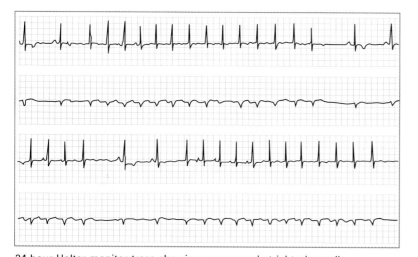

24 hour Holter monitor trace showing paroxysmal atrial tachycardia.

Electrocardiographic diagnosis of atrial tachycardia

- No sawtoothed appearance
- Extrasystolic focus separate from atrioventricular node
- Abnormally shaped P waves at a regular rate, 120–250 beats/min; atrial activity best seen in V1 lead
- Narrow QRS complexes unless conduction defect pre-exists

Junctional tachycardias

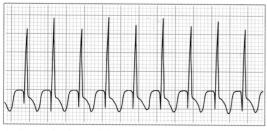

Atrioventricular nodal re-entrant tachycardia.

Atrioventricular nodal re-entrant tachycardia

This requires the presence of a micro re-entrant circuit within the atrioventricular node, commonly with a slow antegrade limb and a fast retrograde limb. A typical electrocardiogram shows the P wave buried in the QRS complex.

Atrioventricular re-entrant tachycardia

This requires the presence of an accessory pathway remote from the atrioventricular node, providing a second connection between the atria and ventricles. The arrhythmia therefore results from the repeated circulation of an electrical impulse between the atria and ventricles. This impulse is usually conducted slowly from the atria to ventricles via the atrioventricular node and then rapidly re-enters the atria via the additional pathway.

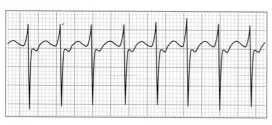

Atrioventricular re-entrant tachycardia.

Diagnosis of atrioventricular re-entrant tachycardia

- Structural heart disease usually absent
- Regular ventricular response
- Atrial activity seen as inverted P wave in the ST segment after each QRS complex
- P waves may be concealed by superimposed terminal portion of the QRS complex
- QRS complexes are narrow and regular, 130–250 beats/min

An accessory pathway on the conventional 12 lead electrocardiogram may be evident as a short PR interval with (as in the Wolff-Parkinson-White syndrome) or without (as in the Lown-Ganong-Levine syndrome) a δ wave.

Sick sinus syndrome

Electrocardiographic diagnosis of sick sinus syndrome

- Inappropriate sinus bradycardia
- Sinus pauses or arrest
- Sinus exit block
- Bradycardias may alternate with tachyarrhythmias, especially:
  Slow and fast atrial fibrillation
  Atrial flutter
  Atrial tachycardia (resulting in the "tachy-brady" syndrome)

The sick sinus syndrome is common, especially in the elderly. It is produced by idiopathic degeneration of the sinoatrial node, resulting in impaired function of the sinus node or sinoatrial conduction. The main problem is the development of bradycardias—for example, sinus bradycardia or episodes of sinus arrest. The syndrome is often associated with various atrial tachyarrhythmias, including atrial fibrillation, atrial flutter, and atrial tachycardia. It may be asymptomatic or have non-specific symptoms, such as dizziness, palpitations, fatigue, syncope, and even sudden death. Using drugs such as digoxin, β blockers, and calcium antagonists may induce or exacerbate symptoms in these patients.

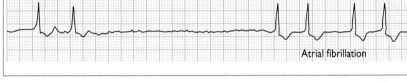

Sinus bradycardia   Pause

Atrial fibrillation

24 hour Holter trace showing sinus bradycardia, pauses, and paroxysmal atrial fibrillation in patient with sick sinus syndrome.

The sick sinus syndrome often becomes evident after a paroxysmal tachycardia (with a depression of sinus node automaticity) leading to sinus arrest or sinus bradycardia. In addition, an atrial tachyarrhythmia may start as an escape rhythm in an underlying bradyarrhythmia—for example, sinus bradycardia or sinus arrest. Such alternation of tachycardias with bradycardias is commonly referred to as the "tachy-brady" syndrome. Abnormal atrioventricular conduction may also coexist in such patients.

Key reference

Zipes DP. Specific arrhythmias: diagnosis and treatment. In: Braunwald E, ed. *Heart disease. A textbook of cardiovascular medicine*, 4th ed. Philadelphia: W B Saunders, 1992; 667–725.

This condition must therefore be considered before antiarrhythmic drug treatment or general anaesthesia is given to any patient with atrial fibrillation and a history of syncope or dizziness. In addition, if an underlying sick sinus syndrome exists then direct current cardioversion of atrial fibrillation may result in asystole and should be covered by a temporary pacemaker. Permanent pacemaker therapy (using an atrial or dual chamber system, depending on atrioventricular conduction) may be successful in such patients, reducing arrhythmias and heart failure and improving prognosis.

4 INVESTIGATION AND NON-DRUG MANAGEMENT OF ATRIAL FIBRILLATION

Gregory Y H Lip, S P Singh, R D S Watson

When a new patient apparently has atrial fibrillation

Is it atrial fibrillation?

Why did the patient develop it? (What is the underlying cause?)

Why does the patient have it now? (Are any precipitating factors present?)

Certain points should be considered when deciding how to manage patients with atrial fibrillation. Firstly, is the diagnosis of atrial fibrillation certain? It is also important to distinguish between chronic and paroxysmal atrial fibrillation as the two conditions have to be managed differently. Secondly, the underlying aetiological or predisposing factor should be sought. Finally, in acute presentations of atrial fibrillation the presence of any acute precipitating factors—for example, infection—should be considered.

Investigations

Diagnosing and assessing atrial fibrillation

Recording of patient's history and clinical features—for example, paroxysmal atrial fibrillation

Documentation of the arrhythmia—for example, with a 24 hour Holter monitor

Echocardiography, especially in young patients

Exercise testing if ischaemic heart disease is present (caution needed in interpreting result if patient is taking digoxin)

The investigation of a patient with atrial fibrillation requires taking a careful clinical history (including medical history), with emphasis on certain clinical features—for example, whether the symptoms are sustained or intermittent and whether any complications, such as heart failure, stroke, or thromboembolism, are present. At the first consultation basic blood tests should be done, including full blood count and tests of renal function, electrolytes, and thyroid function.

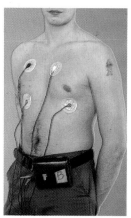

Demonstration of 24 hour Holter monitor.

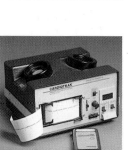

Cardiomemo machine for monitoring patients with intermittent symptoms.

Electrocardiography

The arrhythmia should then be documented, firstly with a conventional 12 lead electrocardiogram. This may provide a clue to the aetiology or electrophysiological features that may cause arrhythmias—for example, ischaemic heart disease (previous myocardial infarction), left ventricular hypertrophy, or a pre-excitation syndrome (δ wave in the Wolff-Parkinson-White syndrome if in sinus rhythm).

A 24 hour Holter monitor may be needed to document paroxysmal atrial fibrillation or the sick sinus syndrome. This investigation is unlikely to be rewarding, however, in patients who have only intermittent and infrequent symptoms such as palpitations. In such patients, a "cardiomemo" (or "transtelephonic event monitor") may be preferred. This device allows an electrocardiographic trace to be transmitted via a telephone; the patient may thus "record" an electrocardiogram during an episode of palpitations. Cardiomemos are fairly cheap, simple to use, and may even be used by general practitioners.

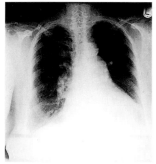

Chest radiograph of patient with atrial septal defect showing cardiomegaly, prominent hila, and pulmonary plethora.

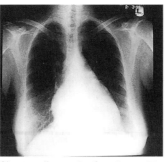

Chest radiograph of patient with mitral stenosis showing straight left heart border, with prominent left atrial appendage and dilated left atrium resulting in a "double contour" next to the right heart border.

Chest radiography

A chest *x* ray examination is useful in most patients with atrial fibrillation. In a young patient it may provide a clue to congenital heart disease, such as atrial septal defect. In an older patient a chest *x* ray film can give information on the size of the heart and whether the patient has heart failure.

Echocardiographic and clinical predictors of stroke in atrial fibrillation

- Independent transthoracic echocardiographic predictors of stroke in patients with atrial fibrillation include left ventricular dysfunction and dilated left atrium:

Echocardiographic finding	Relative risk
Global left ventricular dysfunction	2·6
Dilated left atrium on M mode:	
2·4 cm/m² (left atrium = 4·7)	1·6
2·9 cm/m² (left atrium = 5·7)	2·7

- Clinical risk factors include a history of hypertension, recent (within three months) congestive heart failure, and previous cerebrovascular event (stroke or transient ischaemic attack)

- Percentage risk stratification (per year) for stroke and thromboembolism on the basis of clinical and echocardiographic risk factors:

    1·0 (for patients with no risk factors)
    6·0 (one risk factor)
    18·6 (two or three risk factors)

Echocardiography

Most cardiologists request an echocardiogram for patients with atrial fibrillation. In most patients echocardiography helps to diagnose structural heart disease (including valvar heart disease) and to document left ventricular function.

Echocardiography also complements clinical predictors of the risk of stroke in atrial fibrillation, and may therefore refine risk stratification.

Echocardiography may help to establish the likelihood of successful cardioversion to sinus rhythm—for example, poor left ventricular function is an unfavourable sign. Recently, transoesophageal echocardiography has provided a means of identifying left atrial appendage thrombi, especially if a mitral prosthetic valve is in situ.

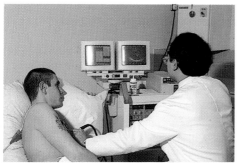

Demonstration of echocardiography.

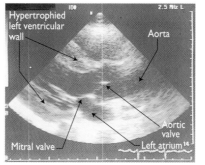

Two dimensional echocardiogram showing left ventricular hypertrophy.

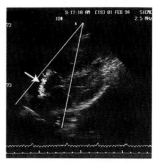

Echocardiogram showing atrial septal defect. Arrow shows colour Doppler signal of blood flow through defect.

Role of echocardiography

To refine the thromboembolic risk stratification in patients unsuitable for cardioversion (echocardiography may also help to determine which patients need warfarin or aspirin)

To identify patients who might be suitable for cardioversion to sinus rhythm

To help to classify patients with "lone" atrial fibrillation

To help to diagnose patients with congenital heart disease, such as an atrial septal defect

To help to exclude intracardiac thrombus, especially in patients with atrial fibrillation and stroke or thromboembolism, and, possibly, before cardioversion (transoesophageal echocardiography is particularly useful for these purposes)

In practice, however, atrial fibrillation is so common in the general population that the resources available for routine echocardiography would be grossly insufficient; the public health issues surrounding the management of atrial fibrillation have so far been largely ignored.

Investigation and non-drug management of atrial fibrillation

Atrial fibrillation—standard investigations

Blood tests
- Full blood count—especially when anticoagulants are being considered
- Urea and electrolytes—to establish baseline and if considering drug treatment (for example, reduced dose of digoxin in renal impairment)
- Thyroid function tests

Electrocardiography, including ambulatory electrocardiography
- 12 lead electrocardiogram
- Possible use of 24 hour Holter monitor—if patient presents with syncope, and paroxysmal atrial fibrillation or the sick sinus syndrome is suspected
- Possibly use of cardiomemo—if symptons are only intermittent and infrequent

Chest radiography

Echocardiography
- Standard transthoracic echocardiography and Doppler ultrasound examination
- Possibly transoesophageal echocardiography if a prosthetic mitral valve is in situ or if endocarditis or atrial thrombi are suspected

---

Exercise testing

Exercise testing is necessary in some patients with ischaemic heart disease and atrial fibrillation to clarify the severity of underlying cardiac ischaemia. Exercise electrocardiograms must be interpreted cautiously, however, if treatment with digoxin is given. Such testing may also have a role in assessing the adequacy of drug treatment in controlling the ventricular response in atrial fibrillation.

Electrophysiology studies

In patients with atrial fibrillation due to a pre-excitation syndrome, referral to a specialist for electrophysiology studies may be needed to document the characteristics of conduction from the atria to the ventricles and the presence of accessory pathways. This may also lead to a "cure" of the condition by transcatheter ablation of the accessory pathway.

Non-drug management

Non-drug treatment

Avoidance of precipitating factors—for example, alcohol

Pacemaker for the sick sinus syndrome

Ablation of an accessory pathway—for example, the Wolff-Parkinson-White syndrome

Ablation of the atrioventricular node and insertion of a permanent pacemaker

Surgery—for example, the "maze" and "corridor" procedures

General measures

General measures—such as asking the patient to reduce his or her caffeine or alcohol intake in cases of paroxysmal atrial fibrillation—should always be considered. Conditions that may benefit from atrial pacing—for example, the sick sinus syndrome—should also be considered. In patients with acute conditions—for example, those who develop atrial fibrillation postoperatively—hypoxia and abnormalities in the electrolytes should be excluded.

It is also important to distinguish between atrial fibrillation and atrial flutter as important differences exist in the management of these two conditions.

Ablation and implantation of pacemaker

In patients with atrial fibrillation and rapid ventricular rates that are poorly controlled by drugs, atrioventricular node and His bundle ablation, and implantation of a permanent pacemaker may be considered. If paroxysmal atrial fibrillation is present as part of the sick sinus syndrome then a permanent pacemaker should be considered. Either an atrial or a dual chamber pacemaker may be used, depending on the integrity of the atrioventricular pathway.

Electrical ablation of the atrioventricular bundle with a transvenous catheter and insertion of a permanent pacemaker was first described by Scheinman and colleagues in 1982. Ablation for arrhythmias is a specialist procedure in which the atrioventricular node is destroyed without surgery, usually by using a high energy radiofrequency current via electrodes on a catheter. Concomitant implantation of a permanent pacemaker is required, however, as ablation of the atrioventricular node results in a complete heart block.

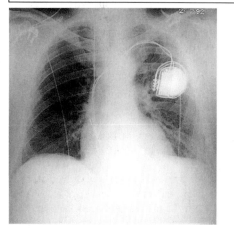

Chest radiograph showing position of dual chamber pacemaker.

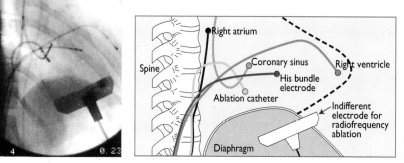

x ray film (and diagram) showing radiofrequency ablation of accessory pathway with electrodes (30° right anterior oblique projection).

The technique results in control of the ventricular rate but sacrifices the physiological pacemaker function of the sinoatrial node. In addition, atrial transport is lost, and, as the risk of thromboembolism remains, anticoagulant treatment is still needed. Electrical ablation is also used in patients with a pre-excitation syndrome secondary to an accessory pathway, in which ablation of the anomalous conducting tissue is performed.

Investigation and non-drug management of atrial fibrillation

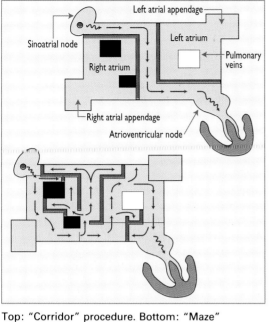

Top: "Corridor" procedure. Bottom: "Maze" procedure. Both procedures have been advocated in patients with atrial fibrillation refractory to medical treatment.

Surgery

Surgery for atrial fibrillation has been advocated for treatment of atrial fibrillation refractory to medical treatment, but, although effective, it is unlikely (at least in Britain) to be adopted generally except for specific patients.

The two most promising surgical options are the "corridor" and "maze" procedures. The corridor procedure effectively isolates both the left and the right atrium, leaving a strip of myocardium connecting the sinus node to the atrioventricular node. This procedure does not prevent atrial fibrillation but isolates the fibrillating atria. Although a 70% "cure" rate is reported, sequential atrioventricular contraction is not restored (with the consequent haemodynamic effects), and the risk of thromboembolism remains.

The maze procedure is intended to prevent atrial fibrillation completely by channelling the atrial activation between a series of incisions. This procedure therefore restores coordinated atrial as well as ventricular electrical activity, permitting atrial transport with good haemodynamic results and low thromboembolic risk.

Initial reports from both these procedures are encouraging, but postoperative implantation of a pacemaker may still be necessary, and the procedure is irreversible.

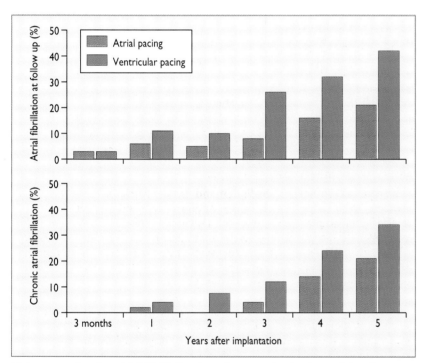

Histograms showing atrial fibrillation in patients randomised to atrial and ventricular pacing in sick sinus syndrome. Chronic atrial fibrillation was defined as atrial fibrillation at two consecutive visits.

Management of sick sinus syndrome

In the presence of symptomatic bradyarrhythmias, permanent pacing is indicated. Evidence exists that simple ventricular pacing systems may result in an increase in the incidence of permanent and paroxysmal atrial fibrillation, hypotension (with a fall of cardiac output of up to one third), thromboembolic events (stroke or peripheral artery embolus), congestive heart failure, and worsened prognosis. In contrast, regular atrial pacing, either alone or combined with ventricular pacing, is often effective in preventing paroxysmal atrial fibrillation associated with the "tachy-brady syndrome" (alternating tachycardia and bradycardia), perhaps by stabilising the atrium electrically, and can therefore improve the overall prognosis. In addition, atrial pacing preserves the normal sequence of cardiac chamber activation.

Patients with the sick sinus syndrome also seem to be at increased thromboembolic risk, and this is thought to be associated with the tachy-brady syndrome. Such patients therefore also need formal anticoagulation.

Key references

Brugada P, Gürsoy S, Brugada J, Andries E. Investigation of palpitations. *Lancet* 1993;**341**:1254–8.
Wagshal AB, Pires LA, Huang SKS. Management of cardiac arrhythmias with radiofrequency of catheter ablation. *Arch Intern Med* 1995;**155**:137–47
McComb JM. Surgery for atrial fibrillation. *Br Heart J* 1994;**71**:501–3.

The illustrations are adapted, with permission of the journals or copyright holders, from: Cox *et al.* The surgical treatment of atrial fibrillation. Development of a definitive surgical procedure. *J Thorac Cardiovasc Surg* 1991;**101**:569–83 (diagrams of the corridor and maze procedures); and Andersen *et al.* Prospective randomised trial of atrial versus ventricular pacing in sick-sinus syndrome. *Lancet* 1994;**344**:1523–8 (graphs). The source of the data in the box of echocardiographic and clinical predictors of stroke is the Stroke Prevention in Atrial Fibrillation Investigators, *Ann Intern Med* 1992;**116**:6–12.

5 DRUGS FOR ATRIAL FIBRILLATION

Gregory Y H Lip, Robert D S Watson, Shyam P Singh

Vaughan-Williams classification of antiarrhythmic drugs

- Class I—Membrane-stabilising agents (fast sodium channel blockers)
  Class Ia—Blocks sodium channel and delays repolarisation, increasing duration of action potential (for example, quinidine, disopyramide, procainamide)
  Class Ib—Blocks sodium channel and accelerates repolarisation, decreasing duration of action potential (for example, lignocaine, phenytoin)
  Class Ic—Blocks sodium channel, with little effect on repolarisation (for example, flecainide, propafenone)
- Class II—β Adrenoceptor blockers
  For example, atenolol, metoprolol
- Class III—Drugs increasing duration of action potential
  For example, amiodarone, bretylium, sotalol (also has class II activity)
- Class IV—Calcium channel blockers
  For example, verapamil, diltiazem

An approach to drug management of atrial fibrillation

Paroxysmal atrial fibrillation
- Consider drugs for preventation of paroxysms and maintenance of sinus rhythm
- Consider treatment with antithrombotic drugs

Chronic atrial fibrillation
- What is the objective of management? Consider cardioversion to sinus rhythm or heart rate control
- Cardioversion: Is the patient taking anticoagulants? Have antiarrhythmic drugs to maintain sinus rhythm after cardioversion been considered?
- Heart rate control: Has the appropriate drug been chosen? Has treatment with antithrombotic drugs been considered?

One of the most important principles of using antiarrhythmic drugs for controlling any arrhythmia is to treat only patients who are symptomatic, have malignant arrhythmias (such as ventricular fibrillation), or are haemodynamically compromised (for example, with hypotension or heart failure). If a patient has only mild and infrequent symptoms, treatment with antiarrhythmic drugs should be avoided. This strategy is justified by evidence of substantial morbidity associated with such treatment and worsened long term prognosis, particularly if class I agents are used. Many antiarrhythmic drugs also depress cardiac function and may precipitate heart failure, and most can aggravate or cause an arrhythmia (arrhythmogenesis or proarrhythmic effect).

Antiarrhythmic drugs can be used for rate control of chronic atrial fibrillation, cardioversion of atrial fibrillation to sinus rhythm, maintenance of sinus rhythm after cardioversion, and control of symptoms. Furthermore, these drugs may be used as prophylaxis in paroxysmal atrial fibrillation. Recent evidence also suggests antithrombotic prophylaxis with warfarin or aspirin should be given. Prescribing habits for atrial fibrillation, however, vary greatly, perhaps reflecting uncertainty about what the best drug is and a lack of scientific evidence from controlled trials.

Digoxin

Digoxin toxicity

Is common in elderly people

May occur with renal impairment

May occur with electrolyte abnormalities (for example, after use of diuretics resulting in hypokalaemia)

May result from interaction with other drugs (for example, quinidine, amiodarone)

Should be anticipated by monitoring of drug levels and serum electrolytes

---

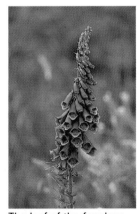

The leaf of the foxglove (*Digitalis purpurea*) contains digitoxin. Most commercial digoxin is now obtained from *Digitalis lanata*.

Digoxin remains the most commonly prescribed antiarrhythmic drug in patients with atrial fibrillation. It is useful in controlling the resting ventricular rate in atrial fibrillation. It has limited value, however, in patients with an accessory pathway (and may even accelerate the ventricular response). In addition, digoxin poorly controls the ventricular response in exercise and in conditions of high sympathetic drive. In such conditions, adequate rate control requires the concomitant use of a β blocker or calcium antagonist with actions at the atrioventricular node, such as verapamil or diltiazem.

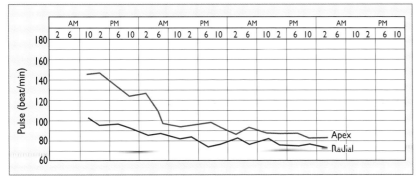

Ward observation chart showing apex-radial pulse deficit in patient with atrial fibrillation who had been given digoxin. This illustrates the relatively slow onset of action of digoxin in achieving satisfactory rate control.

Conditions for resistance of atrial fibrillation to digoxin

Patient is not taking tablets

Accessory pathway is present (for example, the Wolff-Parkinson-White syndrome)

Thyrotoxicosis

Poor left ventricular function

Respiratory disease (including cor pulmonale, pleural effusion, and lung cancer)

Metabolic and electrolyte abnormalities, hypoxia

Drug treatment in patients with paroxysmal atrial fibrillation

Avoid digoxin

If no contraindications try sotalol

Alternatively, try propafenone or other class I drug (but not if cardiac impairment is present)

If poor left ventricular function is present use amiodarone as first choice

---

Drugs for atrial fibrillation

Digoxin has a relatively slow onset of action in achieving a satisfactory ventricular rate response in a patient with fast atrial fibrillation. Although intravenous digoxin does begin to work sooner (less than 30 minutes) than oral digoxin (about 30–60 minutes, or more), it does not work instantaneously. In fact, oral digitalisation with a loading dose still takes several hours to have its maximum effect in slowing the rate and caution is necessary in elderly patients or those with renal impairment.

Digoxin is commonly prescribed in paroxysmal atrial fibrillation both to suppress the arrhythmia and to control the initial heart rate if any such paroxysms occur. But, although it remains an effective treatment for chronic atrial fibrillation, it may be detrimental in paroxysmal atrial fibrillation. There is also no evidence that digoxin is useful for cardioversion of atrial fibrillation to sinus rhythm, or maintaining sinus rhythm after cardioversion.

Clinical evidence has shown that paroxysms of atrial fibrillation occur more frequently and for appreciably longer in patients receiving digoxin. Furthermore, the initial heart rate in such patients is poorly controlled. The mechanism behind this poor control is unclear. Digoxin increases vagal tone, moderating the speed of atrioventricular conduction, and also reduces the atrial refractory period. This latter property may paradoxically render the atrium more susceptible to fibrillation and may reduce or even prevent the chance of reversion to sinus rhythm.

Verapamil and diltiazem

Drawbacks of verapamil

- Verapamil (a class IV drug) is associated with a much lower rate of conversion to sinus rhythm than drugs in class III (for example, amiodarone, sotalol) or class I (for example, flecainide, propafenone)
- It is ineffective in controlling paroxysmal atrial fibrillation
- Giving verapamil to patients with underlying Wolff-Parkinson-White syndrome may lead to serious adverse effects, including ventricular fibrillation and severe haemodynamic impairment. This is due to poor control of very fast ventricular rates in response to electrical impulses passing down the accessory pathway, as the atrioventricular node is blocked by verapamil

Another commonly prescribed drug, verapamil, increases atrioventricular block and the effective refractory period of the atrioventricular node. This results in control of the ventricular rate in sustained atrial fibrillation and may lead to much improved exercise capacity. Verapamil is therefore useful in controlling the ventricular response in atrial fibrillation, both at rest and with exercise. Diltiazem acts in a similar way to verapamil and is a popular alternative in North America.

Class I antiarrhythmic drugs

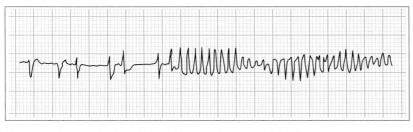

Torsades des pointes in patient taking quinidine for atrial fibrillation.

Class I antiarrhythmic drugs remain popular for atrial fibrillation, especially in North America. Many class I agents, however, have adverse side effects, including proarrhythmic properties, associated with prolongation of the QT interval and torsades des pointes (a polymorphic ventricular tachycardia). Many of these drugs should therefore be started in hospital under medical supervision.

Drugs for atrial fibrillation

It is important, however, to distinguish between atrial fibrillation and flutter, as the use of a class I agent in patients with atrial flutter may accelerate the ventricular response with a 1:1 atrioventricular conduction. This may be due partly to the slowing in atrial rate and the anticholinergic effects (especially with disopyramide and quinidine), which result in an increase in atrioventricular conduction. Therefore if class I agents are given in atrial flutter then digoxin, β blockers, or verapamil should be given alongside to avoid the potential for the accelerated atrioventricular conduction.

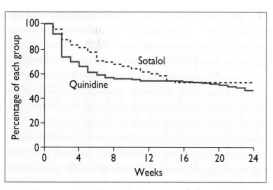

Efficacy of quinidine in maintaining sinus rhythm after cardioversion.

Class Ia

Quinidine is used often, especially in North America, for maintaining sinus rhythm after cardioversion or for reducing the frequency of paroxysmal atrial fibrillation. This strategy is supported by a meta-analysis of six controlled trials that showed that patients treated with quinidine were less likely to have a recurrence of atrial fibrillation. Importantly, however, this analysis also showed an excess of mortality for the treated group. Quinidine also interacts with digoxin and is associated with serious side effects, such as polymorphic ventricular tachycardia, quinidine syncope, blood dyscrasias, and cinchonism.

Disopyramide may also prevent recurrences of atrial fibrillation, but its effects are inconsistent. It is also poorly tolerated, particularly in elderly people and those with glaucoma and prostatism, primarily because of its profound anticholinergic properties. Procainamide also shares some electrophysiological properties with quinidine and disopyramide, but no placebo controlled studies of this drug have been carried out.

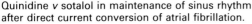

Quinidine *v* sotalol in maintenance of sinus rhythm after direct current conversion of atrial fibrillation.

Class Ic

By contrast, class Ic antiarrhythmic drugs, such as flecainide and propafenone, have been well investigated. They have potent effects on conduction within cardiac cell membranes and lengthen the PR interval and QRS complex in the electrocardiogram. Flecainide has been shown to be effective in preventing recurrences of atrial fibrillation in up to 60% of patients but does not limit the ventricular response. Adverse effects with flecainide have been reported in up to 74% of patients, but these effects were mostly tolerable. Nevertheless, doubts about the safety of flecainide have been raised by the Cardiac Arrhythmia Suppression Trial, in which patients (with previous myocardial infarction) given flecainide for ventricular arrhythmias had a worsened prognosis (with about a threefold increase in mortality).

Although limited information exists, the safety record in patients with atrial arrhythmias may be more favourable. Flecainide may be used with caution in patients with atrial fibrillation without evidence of ischaemic heart disease or ventricular dysfunction, especially to control paroxysmal atrial fibrillation, achieve pharmacological cardioversion, or to control atrial fibrillation associated with the Wolff-Parkinson-White syndrome. Current recommendations in the *British National Formulary* are that treatment with these drugs should be started in hospital under supervision.

Propafenone may also be effective in paroxysmal atrial fibrillation. This is particularly pertinent in view of its inherent rate limiting (class II) properties, permitting potentially greater ventricular rate control. In paroxysmal atrial fibrillation flecainide may be more effective than propafenone in converting patients to sinus rhythm (90% *v* 55% conversion rate respectively). Propafenone and solatol (which also has class III activity), however, are equally effective in maintaining sinus rhythm in patients with recurrent atrial fibrillation.

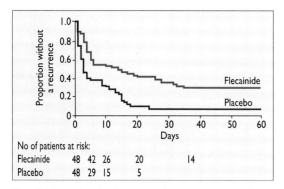

Flecainide *v* placebo in prevention of symptomatic recurrences of paroxysmal atrial fibrillation.

Class III antiarrhythmic drugs

Useful drug options in various clinical situations

Atrial fibrillation in hypertensive patient
Calcium antagonist (for example, verapamil, diltiazem)

Atrial fibrillation and thyroid disease
Non-specific β blocker (for example propranolol)

Atrial fibrillation and ischaemic heart disease
β Blocker if possible (otherwise diltiazem, verapamil)

Heart failure and poor cardiac function
Digoxin or possibly amiodarone

Atrial fibrillation and hypertrophic cardiomyopathy
β Blockers or calcium antagonists

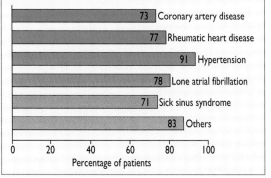

Success of amiodarone in maintaining sinus rhythm in patients with atrial fibrillation with respect to underlying aetiology.

A stepped care approach to drugs for rate control in chronic atrial fibrillation

- Try digoxin first
- If unsuccessful add or substitute verapamil, diltiazem, or β blocker
- If still unsuccessful consider adding or substituting propafenone, flecainide, or amiodarone
- Referral to specialist may be indicated in difficult cases

Sotalol, another commonly prescribed drug, combines the antiarrhythmic effects of drugs in both class II (blockade) and class III (prolongation of repolarisation). This second property is thought to be mainly due to the dextro (D) isomer of the sotalol compound. Little evidence exists, however, for the efficacy of sotalol specifically in paroxysmal atrial fibrillation, although the evidence suggests that sotalol is effective in maintaining sinus rhythm post-cardioversion. Sotalol seems effective in controlling the ventricular response in atrial fibrillation, thus permitting rate control, without the need for other drugs, such as digoxin. As sotalol has β blocker activity, it may also be useful in patients with concomitant ischaemic heart disease and hypertension.

Amiodarone is a very effective drug for treating atrial fibrillation, but its use has to be moderated because of its common side effects, although serious side effects do not often occur with maintenance doses of 200 mg or less. Side effects of amiodarone include photosensitivity and skin rashes, hepatic dysfunction or hepatitis, pulmonary fibrosis, neuromyopathy, and thyroid disorders. These side effects are more common with higher doses of amiodarone and with prolonged treatment, although some may be reversible on withdrawal of the drug. Nevertheless, amiodarone is particularly useful in atrial fibrillation for treating patients refractory to other measures, and low doses of 200 mg/day (often much less than doses needed for controlling ventricular arrhythmias, which require 400 mg/day or more) may be effective with little risk of side effects.

Amiodarone has also been shown to be highly effective in converting atrial fibrillation to sinus rhythm and to be capable of maintaining sinus rhythm long term. It also seems more effective than either verapamil or quinidine and is highly effective in controlling symptoms, possibly moderating the ventricular response even if an attack occurs. Amiodarone may have a particular role in patients with arrhythmias and severe impairment of left ventricular function. It can be given orally (when it has a slow onset of action related to a prolonged half-life of weeks) or intravenously for more rapid effect. The use of a rapid loading regimen of intravenous amiodarone to suppress paroxysmal atrial fibrillation is, however, seldom indicated. Care should also be taken with amiodarone as it can substantially increase the plasma concentration of digoxin, thus leading to potential toxicity. It also commonly leads to overanticoagulation in patients taking warfarin, perhaps by a hepatic interaction.

Key references

Channer KS. The drug treatment of atrial fibrillation. *Br J Clin Pharmacol* 1991;**32**:267–73.
Cowan JC. Antiarrhythmic drugs in the management of atrial fibrillation. *Br Heart J* 1993;**70**:304–6
Lip GYH, Metcalfe MJ, Rae AP. Management of paroxysmal atrial fibrillation. *Q J Med* 1993;**86**:467–72.
Reiffel JA, Estes NAM, Waldo AL, Prystowsky EN, DiBianco R. A consensus report on antiarrhythmic drug use. *Clin Cardiol* 1994;**17**:103–16.

The histograms were adapted, with permission, from Coplen *et al, Circulation* 1990;**82**:1106–16 (efficacy of quinidine after cardioversion); Juul-Möller *et al, Circulation* 1990;**82**:1932–9 (solatol *v* quinidine); Anderson *et al, Circulation* 1989;**80**:1557–70 (flecainide); and Gold *et al, Am J Cardiol* 1986;**57**:124–7 (amiodarone). The information in the box of the Vaughan-Williams classification is adapted from Singh BN, Vaughan Williams EM. Classification of antiarrhythmic drugs. In: Sandor E *et al*, ed. *Symposium on cardiac arrhythmias.* Sodertalje: AB Astra, 1970.

6 ANTITHROMBOTIC TREATMENT FOR ATRIAL FIBRILLATION

Gregory Y H Lip, Gordon D O Lowe

> **Atrial fibrillation is an important risk factor for stroke, and antithrombotic treatment should be considered in most patients with this arrhythmia**

Although atrial fibrillation has long been recognised as a risk factor for thromboembolic events, preventive treatment has, until recently, been both empirical and controversial. Only in the past few years have antithrombotic drugs been proved by prospective clinical studies to be effective against strokes in atrial fibrillation.

Atrial fibrillation and thromboembolism

> **Non-rheumatic atrial fibrillation and stroke**
>
> - Non-rheumatic atrial fibrillation has been associated with a fivefold increase in the risk of ischaemia stroke
> - The yearly risk is 5–7%, increasing with age
> - Computed tomography studies have shown that silent ischaemic cerebral infarction is present in 26% of patients with non-rheumatic atrial fibrillation

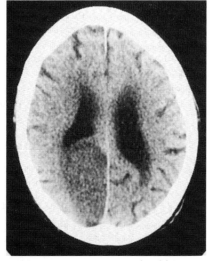

Computed tomogram showing large thrombotic stroke.

The pathophysiological mechanism for thromboembolism seems to be the disturbed blood flow in the fibrillating left atrium, which predisposes to the formation of thrombi and arterial embolism, especially in the presence of underlying heart disease. About 15–20% of patients who have an acute stroke have atrial fibrillation at the time of their stroke; mortality is one and a half to three times higher in those patients than in patients with sinus rhythm at the time of stroke.

Underlying heart disease

Underlying heart disease—including valvar and hypertensive heart disease, an enlarged left atrium, and poor left ventricular function—is a contributory risk factor for stroke and thromboembolism in atrial fibrillation. The risk of thromboembolism in atrial fibrillation is 18 times greater if rheumatic heart disease is present. In the stroke prevention in atrial fibrillation study, the presence of recent (within three months) congestive heart failure and left ventricular dysfunction on echocardiography also contributed to an increased risk of thromboembolism in atrial fibrillation. This is consistent with the observation that thromboembolism is a common cause of death in patients with congestive heart failure, occurring in up to 30% of patients, which is partly preventable by anticoagulation.

Left atrial enlargement and spontaneous echo contrast

An enlarged left atrium may contribute to an increased risk of atrial thrombi and thromboembolism in patients with atrial fibrillation. An enlarged left atrium has also been associated with "spontaneous echo contrast" on transoesophageal echocardiography—a smoke-like appearance of blood in the atria, suggesting sluggish flow. It is associated with dilated left atria, intracardiac thrombi, thromboembolism, stroke, abnormal rheology, and coagulation.

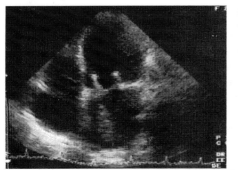
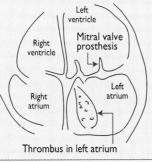

Echocardiogram (with diagram) showing prosthetic mitral valve and thrombus in left atrium.

Labels: Left ventricle, Right ventricle, Mitral valve prosthesis, Right atrium, Left atrium, Thrombus in left atrium

Previous cerebrovascular disease or thromboembolism

A history of stroke, transient ischaemic attack, or other embolic events adds to the risk of stroke and mortality in atrial fibrillation. The pooled analysis by the Atrial Fibrillation Investigators showed that a previous stroke or transient ischaemic attack was an independent risk factor for further strokes. Using warfarin in such patients reduced the annual rate of stroke from 12% a year to 5%.

Paroxysmal and chronic atrial fibrillation and stroke risk

- A third of patients with paroxysmal atrial fibrillation develop chronic atrial fibrillation over two to three years
- The risk of stroke is highest during the first months after the initial diagnosis of atrial fibrillation or immediately after a transition from paroxysmal to chronic atrial fibrillation
- The recent pooled analysis by the Atrial Fibrillation Investigators suggested that patients with paroxysmal atrial fibrillation and chronic atrial fibrillation had a similar risk of stroke, although the length of time a patient was in atrial fibrillation had no discernible effect on the risk

---

Paroxysmal atrial fibrillation may be associated with the sick sinus syndrome, and patients with this condition are at particular risk of stroke and thromboembolism.

In a Glasgow study, among patients admitted with acute severe stroke, those with atrial fibrillation (25%) had a significantly higher hospital mortality than those in sinus rhythm (67% v 44%). This was confirmed in the Oxfordshire community stroke project, in which the 30 day mortality among patients with acute stroke was three times higher than those with atrial fibrillation (17%) than among those in sinus rhythm.

Hypertension and diabetes

A history of hypertension and diabetes add to the risk of stroke in atrial fibrillation. Using warfarin in patients with a history of hypertension or diabetes would reduce the annual rate of stroke respectively from 5–6% to 2% and from 9% to 3%.

Duration and onset of atrial fibrillation

The onset of atrial fibrillation may be related to the imminence of stroke. In the Framingham study, atrial fibrillation was present at the time of stroke in 24% of subjects, and about a third of the strokes associated with atrial fibrillation occurred within six months of onset of the arrhythmia. In addition, a further stroke within six months of the first may be more common in patients with continued atrial fibrillation, although this was not confirmed in the Oxfordshire study.

Many patients with paroxysmal atrial fibrillation go on to develop chronic atrial fibrillation, and thromboembolic complications often occur during the transition.

Clinical trials of warfarin and aspirin prophylaxis

Important stroke prevention trials

AFASAK	Copenhagen atrial fibrillation, aspirin, anticoagulation study
BAATAF	Boston area anticoagulation trial for atrial fibrillation
CAFA	Canadian atrial fibrillation anticoagulation study
EAFT	European atrial fibrillation trial
SPAF	Stroke prevention in atrial fibrillation trial
SPINAF	Stroke prevention in nonrheumatic atrial fibrillation study

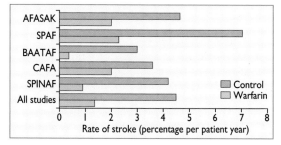

Efficacy of warfarin in atrial fibrillation trials—total risk reduction for all five trials combined is 68% (P<0·001).

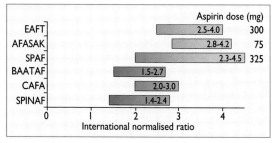

Ranges of international normalised ratios used in atrial fibrillation trials.

Warfarin

In the mid-1980s five randomised prospective clinical trials were independently started to define the value of anticoagulant prophylaxis with warfarin in patients with atrial fibrillation. These five primary prevention studies showed consistent results. Since publication of the results another primary prevention trial (the second stroke prevention in atrial fibrillation study) has been reported, as well as a secondary prevention trial in patients with non-rheumatic atrial fibrillation and a history of transient ischaemic attack or minor stroke (European atrial fibrillation trial).

The pooled analysis of the five primary intervention trials showed that warfarin reduced the annual rate of stroke; led to a similar risk reduction in stroke with residual deficit; reduced mortality by a third; and reduced the rate of the combined adverse outcome (stroke, systemic embolism, or death) by half. The efficacy of warfarin prophylaxis was in fact underestimated because most strokes in patients allocated to warfarin occurred while the patient was not taking his or her warfarin.

The five primary prevention trials used different target therapeutic ranges of the international normalised ratio of the prothrombin time; the target range in all studies was 1·5 to 4·5. The minimum risk of stroke seemed to occur in the range 2·0 to 3·0, which is now accepted as the optimum therapeutic range for warfarin prophylaxis of thromboembolism in all patients except those with older, mechanical prosthetic heart valves and those with recurrent thromboembolism despite warfarin prophylaxis at the range 2·0 to 3·0 (such patients merit higher intensity warfarin (range 3·0 to 4·5)). At present, therefore, a target range of 2·0 to 3·0 can be recommended in the absence of the above indications for high intensity warfarin.

Risk of bleeding with anticoagulation treatment

- Risk of bleeding in patients taking warfarin increases exponentially with an increase in anticoagulant effect, rising from an annual risk of 0·2% with an international normalised ratio of 2·0% to 3·0% with a ratio of 4·0
- Bleeding is most common in patients with unstable anticoagulation control and those with a history of thromboembolism and ranges from 11% to 40%
- Complications related to bleeding may occur often, however, even when the international normalised ratio is within the therapeutic range

---

Does evidence from prevention studies apply to clinical practice?

- The patient population was highly selected—for example, >90% of those screened in many of the studies were excluded from entry
- The rate of patient withdrawal in the studies was often high (19% to 38%)
- Patients in usual clinical practice may have different risks of thromboembolism and bleeding from selected patients participating in trials
- The compliance, and therefore safety, of warfarin may be poorer when it is used in clinical practice than when it is used in carefully selected, well motivated, and closely monitored study participants

---

Further questions on antithrombotic treatment in atrial fibrillation

- What is the efficacy of aspirin (which does not need laboratory monitoring and carries a lower risk of bleeding) compared with warfarin as antithrombotic prophylaxis?
- For which patients with the highest risk of thromboembolism may the risk of bleeding and the monitoring of warfarin prophylaxis be most justified?
- Are there any patients whose risk of thromboembolism is so low that neither aspirin nor warfarin prophylaxis is indicated?

Intracranial haemorrhage is the most feared complication of warfarin prophylaxis. The annual risks of intracranial haemorrhage increased from 0·1% in the controls to 0·3% in patients taking warfarin in the pooled analysis. This risk was associated with an international normalised ratio >3·0 and with uncontrolled hypertension; there was also a non-signifcant association with increasing age. Lower intensity warfarin (for example, target ratio 1·5 to 2·5) is currently being compared with higher intensity warfarin in the third stroke prevention in atrial fibrillation study; meanwhile some physicians use low intensity warfarin in patients for whom the usual target range of 2·0 to 3·0 is judged to carry an unacceptable risk of bleeding.

Despite the convincing evidence from the pooled analysis of randomised trials that warfarin prophylaxis is highly effective and seems to outweigh substantially the risk of intracranial bleeding (as well as other types of major bleeding), the efficacy of warfarin in clinical trials may not be reproduced in practice. This is due to the high selection of patients in these studies.

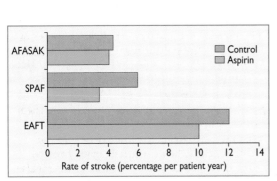

Efficacy of aspirin in atrial fibrillation trials—total risk reduction for all three trials combined is 21% (P = 0·04).

Aspirin

Aspirin has been evaluated as primary prophylaxis of systemic thromboembolism—in two randomised trials compared with no antithrombotic treatment and in one compared with warfarin: aspirin was only about half as effective as warfarin, with a 36% decrease in risk of stroke. Aspirin prophylaxis had no significant effect on stroke with residual deficit or mortality; but there was a 28% decrease in the rate of the combined outcome of stroke, systemic embolism, or death.

The annual risk of stroke seems low, however, in patients at moderate risk treated with aspirin, and aspirin is simpler to monitor and has a lower risk of bleeding. Aspirin was less effective than warfarin, however, when given as secondary prophylaxis in patients with previous stroke or transient ischaemic attack, who have a higher risk of thromboembolism.

Risk of stroke in patients with atrial fibrillation, stratified by risk, with and without antithrombotic prophylaxis. Values are percentages per patient per year

Risk	No prophylaxis	Asprin	Warfarin
High:			
Previous stroke or transient ischaemic attack	12	10	4–5
Age ⩾75, other clinical risk factors*	8	4–5	1–2
Moderate:			
Age <65, other clinical risk factors*			
Age 65–74	4	1–3	1–2
Age ⩾75, no clinical risk factors			
Low:			
Age <65, no clinical risk factors	1	<1	<1

* Such as diabetes and hypertension.

Risk stratification for warfarin, aspirin, or no antithrombotic prophylaxis

The relative risk of stroke in people with non-rheumatic atrial fibrillation (and hence the absolute benefits of antithrombotic prophylaxis with warfarin or aspirin) varies greatly with the presence of risk factors for thromboembolism. The risk of stroke in non-rheumatic atrial fibrillation seems similar in men and women, and in people with continuous atrial fibrillation and in those with paroxysmal atrial fibrillation.

Identifying patients with atrial fibrillation at high risk of stroke and thromboembolism

- Many such patients may be unrecognised and undiagnosed in the community, with few or no symptoms
- Formal screening for atrial fibrillation in primary care should be considered
- Careful clinical history is needed to identify those with important risk factors
- Echocardiography may be a further tool in thromboembolic risk stratification
- Recent studies suggest that a "hypercoagulable" state exists in patients with atrial fibrillation

The highest risk of stroke (annual risk 12%) is in people with previous transient ischaemic attack or stroke. Warfarin is more effective in absolute terms as secondary prophylaxis than as primary prophylaxis and also seems more effective than aspirin. In addition to a history of thromboembolism, other independent risk factors for thromboembolism are increasing age (especially age >75 years), diabetes mellitus, and history of hypertension. These high risk patients should be considered for anticoagulation with warfarin.

A moderate risk of stroke (annual risk 4%) exists in people with non-rheumatic atrial fibrillation, without previous embolism, who are (a) aged under 65 years with a history of diabetes or hypertension; (b) aged 65-74 (with or without a history of diabetes or hypertension); or (c) aged 75 years or more with no history of diabetes or hypertension. In such people aspirin seems as effective as warfarin (reducing the annual risk of stroke to 1% to 3%).

A low risk of stroke (annual risk 1%) exists in people with non-rheumatic atrial fibrillation who are aged under 65 years with no history of embolism, hypertension, or diabetes. In such people antithrombotic prophylaxis with either aspirin or warfarin does not seem warranted unless some other indication coexists.

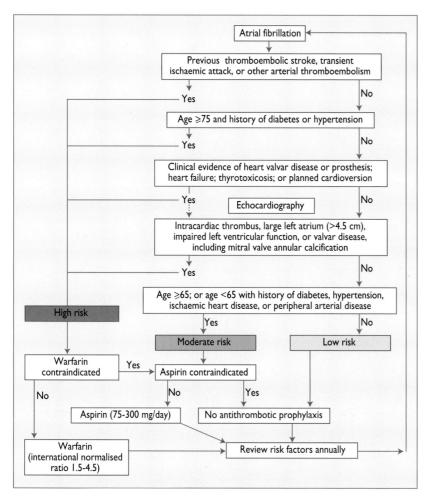

Algorithm for risk stratification and selection of prophylaxis in atrial fibrillation.

Echocardiography may complement the clinical risk stratification of risk of stroke in atrial fibrillation, although the precise contribution in non-rheumatic atrial fibrillation is uncertain (echocardiographic data were not included in the pooled analysis of the Atrial Fibrillation Investigators). There is an increase in risk of stroke, however, with a large left atrium, impaired left ventricular function, or calcification of the mitral valve. An increased risk of systemic embolism has also been observed in patients with atrial fibrillation associated with heart valve disease (for example, rheumatic heart disease), heart valve prosthesis, heart failure, intracardiac thrombus, or thyrotoxicosis. One possible algorithm for risk stratification and selection of prophylaxis in atrial fibrillation is shown.

Factors that may increase risk of bleeding with warfarin

- Age
- Uncontrolled hypertension (systolic blood pressure >180 mm Hg or diastolic blood pressure >100 mm Hg)
- Alcohol excess
- Liver disease
- Poor drug or clinic compliance
- Bleeding lesions (especially gastrointestinal blood loss—for example, peptic ulcer disease—and previous cerebral haemorrhage)
- Tendency to bleeding (including coagulation defects, thrombocytopenia)
- Concomitant use of aspirin with oral anticoagulants

Practical considerations in antithrombotic prophylaxis

Before starting antithrombotic prophylaxis with warfarin or aspirin it is important to balance the risks (especially bleeding) and the benefits in the patient. To minimise the risk of intracranial bleeding with prophylactic warfarin, hypertension should be adequately controlled, and the risks and benefits of warfarin reviewed annually, especially in patients aged over 80.

Antithrombotic treatment for atrial fibrillation

Recommendations by American College of Chest Physicians on starting anticoagulation after acute thromboembolic stroke

- Patients with small or moderate thromboembolic strokes in whom an intracranial bleed is excluded by computed tomography at ≥48 hours:
  Heparin followed by warfarin (international normalised ratio 2·0–3·0)
- Patients with large embolic strokes or uncontrolled hypertension:
  No anticoagulation for 5–14 days because of the increased risk of haemorrhagic transformation
- Patients with non-valvar atrial fibrillation as the presumed cause of thromboembolism:
  Warfarin only (after computed tomography at 48 hours) owing to the low risk of early recurrent thromboembolism

Summary

- Antithrombotic prophylaxis with long term warfarin or aspirin reduces thromboembolic risk in atrial fibrillation
- Identification, risk assessment, and regular review of all patients with atrial fibrillation should be routine in general and hospital practice
- Risk stratification is easily performed on clinical grounds—echocardiography may refine it

Key references

Albers GW. Atrial fibrillation and stroke. *Arch Intern Med* 1994;**154**:1443–8

Atrial Fibrillation Investigators. Risk factors for stroke and efficacy of antithrombotic therapy in atrial fibrillation. *Arch Intern Med* 1994;**154**:1449–57

British Society for Haematology. Guidelines on oral anticoagulation: second edition. *J Clin Pathol* 1990;**43**:177–83

Lip GYH. Does atrial fibrillation confer a hypercoagulable state? *Lancet* 1995;**346**:1313–4

Laupacis A, Albers GW, Dalen JE, Dunn MI, Feinberg W, Jacobson AK. Antithrombotic therapy in atrial fibrillation. *Chest* 1995;**108**(suppl):352–9S.

In patients with acute stroke and atrial fibrillation, intracranial haemorrhage should be excluded—for example, with computed tomography—before starting warfarin. This is important as 11% of patients with haemorrhagic stroke have atrial fibrillation, compared with 18% with stroke due to cerebral infarction. It is important to start anticoagulation at the right time after an acute cardioembolic stroke as there is the risk of haemorrhagic transformation of the cerebral infarct, by bleeding into the infarcted, softened brain.

The graphs showing effectiveness of warfarin and aspirin and the international normalised ratios, have been adapted, with permission, from Albers *et al*, *Arch Intern Med* 1994;**154**:1443-8. The table was adapted, with permission, from Atrial Fibrillation Investigators, *Arch Intern Med* 1994;**154**:1449-57. The recommendations in the box on when to start anticoagulation were adapted from Sherman DG *et al*, *Chest* 1995;**108**(suppl):444–56S.

7 CARDIOVERSION OF ATRIAL FIBRILLATION

Gregory Y H Lip, Robert D S Watson, Shyam P Singh

Suitability for cardioversion

- Recent onset atrial fibrillation
- No structural heart disease, such as mitral valve disease, poor left ventricular function, dilated left atrium
- Successful treatment of any precipitating cause of atrial fibrillation—for example, thyrotoxicosis, chest infection

Cardioversion from atrial fibrillation to sinus rhythm should be considered for suitable patients as an alternative to leaving the patient in a cardiac arrhythmia and treating with drugs. The potential benefits of a return to sinus rhythm are an improvement in wellbeing and exercise capacity; the avoidance of potentially dangerous drug treatment; and a possible reduction in thromboembolic risk.

Electrical cardioversion

Methods of cardioversion

Electrical
- Synchronised external direct current shock
- Transoesophageal
- Internal

Pharmacological
- Class I drugs
- Class III drugs

Electrical cardioversion works by permitting uniform repolarisation and restoring ordered conduction. After the initial asystolic period, the sinoatrial node rapidly resumes its role as cardiac pacemaker, permitting synchronised atrial electrical activity.

External electrical cardioversion with a synchronised direct current shock can be effective in restoring sinus rhythm. The effectiveness of the procedure can range from 20–90% as the procedure is highly influenced by the underlying aetiology—the highest success rates are seen in patients with atrial fibrillation secondary to hyperthyroidism, while the lowest rates are seen in patients with severe mitral regurgitation.

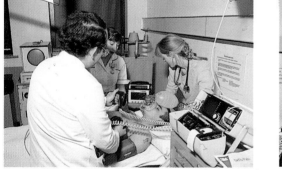

Left: Demonstration of cardioversion under general anaesthetic. Right: Equipment required for cardioversion under general anaesthetic—electrocardiograph, defibrillator to give synchronised shock, pulse oximeter, blood pressure monitor, suction facility, oxygen.

Attention to proper technique for external cardioversion will substantially improve efficacy. The energy requirement and success of external cardioversion are also directly related to the duration of atrial fibrillation, size of the f (fibrillation) waves, and the presence of mitral valve disease (especially if there has been previous valve surgery). Many other factors, however, predict refractoriness to successful cardioversion or unsuccessful maintenance of sinus rhythm.

Transoesophageal cardioversion and internal cardioversion are alternative methods of performing electrical cardioversion, but these are used less often, except in specialist centres.

Pharmacological cardioversion and antiarrythmic treatment

In general, class I and III antiarrhythmic drugs are the most useful agents for pharmacological cardioversion

An alternative to electrical cardioversion is pharmacological cardioversion, especially in patients with atrial fibrillation of recent onset. Drugs that are usually used to maintain sinus rhythm after electrical cardioversion are also effective for pharmacological cardioversion.

Cardioversion of atrial fibrillation

Procedure for cardioversion

Preparation
- Arrange admission for monitoring with electrocardiography—for example, to a coronary care unit
- Ensure electrolytes (especially potassium) are normal
- Ensure anticoagulation is adequate, with an international normalised ratio of 2·0 to 3·0
- If the patient usually takes digoxin and has no evidence of digoxin toxicity the drug may be taken up to the day before cardioversion; if digoxin toxicity is present then serum digoxin concentrations should be checked and cardioversion delayed

Pharmacological cardioversion
- Start infusion of drug—for example, flecainide, amiodarone—under continuous monitoring with electrocardiography

Electrical cardioversion
- Arrange for patient to be fasted
- Give short general anaesthetic to eliminate discomfort associated with the transthoracic shock
- Give synchronised direct current shock: start at 100 J, with intermediate "step-ups", eventually to 360 J
- After the procedure monitor the patient for at least one hour to ensure stability of rhythm and blood pressure

Class I agents

The most commonly used class I drugs are quinidine, flecainide, and propafenone. Quinidine is particularly effective in cardioversion of patients with atrial fibrillation and in maintaining sinus rhythm, but side effects can occur in a fifth of patients, two thirds of whom have to stop taking the drug.

Flecainide and propafenone have a rate of successful cardioversion of 25–55% when given orally. Several studies of flecainide have shown it to have a 92% success rate if given intravenously and to reduce significantly the recurrence of the arrhythmia. The drug has no rate limiting properties, however, and has been reported to cause adverse effects in 74% of patients. Propafenone, another class Ic compound, may be more useful than flecainide in view of its inherent rate limiting properties (as a β blocker), permitting potentially greater ventricular rate control.

Amiodarone

Amiodarone, a class III antiarrhythmic drug, has been shown to be highly effective in the cardioversion of atrial fibrillation, even in previously refractory cases and in maintaining sinus rhythm. An intravenous infusion of amiodarone acts relatively rapidly, restoring sinus rhythm in up to three quarters of cases, making it as effective as electrical cardioversion. In cases of resistant atrial fibrillation, a four week loading of amiodarone (600 mg/day) before cardioversion and a low dose (on average 200 mg/day) maintenance regime after successful cardioversion was effective in achieving cardioversion and sustaining sinus rhythm.

Other drugs

Although occasionally effective in converting atrial fibrillation to sinus rhythm, verapamil has a much lower success rate of conversion than the class I and III antiarrhythmics. Digoxin is no better than placebo for restoring sinus rhythm. Nor does evidence exist that digoxin is effective as prophylaxis against recurring atrial fibrillation after cardioversion. In addition, in patients with recurrent atrial fibrillation, paroxysms of atrial fibrillation occur more frequently, at a faster rate, and for longer in patients receiving digoxin.

Thromboembolism, antithrombotic treatment, and cardioversion

Mechanisms and factors contributing to thromboembolism

Mechanical
- Sudden resumption of mechanical atrial systole may result in the embolisation of any pre-existing clot, which is dislodged by the mechanical effect of a change in cardiac rhythm during cardioversion
- The return of atrial systole and effective atrial contraction after cardioversion may take up to three weeks
- Cardioversion may promote the formation of new thrombi due to transient atrial dysfunction ("stunning")

Duration of atrial fibrillation
- A recently formed, poorly adherent thrombus is more likely to dislodge at the time of cardioversion
- The relationship between duration of atrial fibrillation and thromboembolism is affected by haemodynamic status, atrial size, underlying atrial pathology, and effectiveness of anticoagulation

Left atrial size
- Formation of thrombi is more likely in dilated left atria

Abnormalities in haemorheological function and prothrombotic markers
- Clotting factor levels
- Atrial natriuretic peptide, leading to haemoconcentration, and a raised packed cell volume

Peripheral emboli have been estimated to complicate external cardioversion in 1–3% of cases. Thromboembolism after pharmacological cardioversion probably has similar rates.

The importance of prophylactic anticoagulation in patients with chronic atrial fibrillation is now established. The role of prophylactic anticoagulation to prevent thromboembolism after cardioversion for patients in atrial fibrillation has been clinically examined in several large series, which established that prior anticoagulant treatment was beneficial in attempted cardioversion. The thromboembolic events that occurred in patients who had received anticoagulants were noted predominantly in the first week after cardioversion, suggesting that this is a high risk period.

The dose of warfarin should be adjusted to maintain an international normalised ratio of 2·0 to 3·0, although in patients at high risk of embolism—for example, those with previous thromboembolism or with mechanical prosthetic heart valves—the target is 3·0 to 4·5.

Management after cardioversion

Recommendations of American Association of Chest Physicians for anticoagulation before and after cardioversion

- Warfarin for three weeks before non-emergency cardioversion of atrtial fibrillation of >24–48 hours' duration
- Warfarin for four weeks after cardioversion
- Intravenous heparin followed by warfarin if cardioversion cannot be postponed for three weeks
- Anticoagulants may not be needed for atrial fibrillation of <2 days' duration or for cardioversion of supraventricular tachycardia. Consideration should be given to managing atrial flutter similarly to atrial fibrillation

After successful cardioversion to sinus rhythm it is important to continue with oral anticoagulants. The routine (and optimal) use of antiarrhythmic drugs before and after cardioversion, however, remains controversial. The use of these drugs after cardioversion is to maintain sinus rhythm and prevent recurrence of arrhythmia.

Predictors of refractoriness to cardioversion or unsuccessful maintenance of sinus rhythm

- Age >50 years
- Arrhythmia for >1 year
- Hypertension
- Structural heart disease, including poor cardiac function, valvar disease, previous mitral valve surgery, and other organic heart disease
- No correctable precipitating factor—for example, thyroid disease, infection

Current practice favours maintaining oral anticoagulation after cardioversion. The risk of embolism probably continues even after successful cardioversion as atrial mechanical function may not be restored for several weeks. The optimal duration of anticoagulation is still unclear, although the American Association of Chest Physicians has drawn up recommendations, including the suggestion that warfarin should be continued for four weeks after cardioversion. In patients with a high risk of recurrent atrial fibrillation, however, it may be prudent to continue anticoagulation for longer than four weeks.

Changes after cardioversion of atrial fibrillation

Short term
- Hypotension and bradycardia—bradycardia more common in patients with the sick sinus syndrome and after acute myocardial infarction
- Arrhythmias, usually due to either inadequate synchronisation or digoxin toxicity; ventricular arrhythmias after cardioversion are less common but more serious (ventricular fibrillation is the most common, in about 1% of cases, but is usually reverted by repeat shock)
- Premature beats and conduction disturbances (first degree or second degree atrioventricular block) are also common
- Small rises in creatine kinase concentration may occur with electrical cardioversion, usually from skeletal muscle, and myocardial damage is unlikely
- Raised transient ST segment after cardioversion, usually associated with previous pericardiotomy, age, and diminished long term maintenance of sinus rhythm

Long term
- Reduction in left atrial size
- Improvement in ventricular function and also in some cases cardiac output and exercise or functional capacity due to a combination of a reduction in heart rate and the restoration of atrial systole

Without antiarrhythmic drugs there is a high risk of relapse of atrial fibrillation, with the proportion of patients remaining in sinus rhythm ranging from 69% at one month to 58% at six months, 23% at one year, and 16% at two years. These drugs are most useful during the three months after successful cardioversion. If patients have an identifiable cause of atrial fibrillation that has been corrected—for example, thyrotoxicosis—antiarrhythmic treatment for three months may be sufficient. If patients, however, have no obvious acute precipitating factors and adverse features for recurrence of atrial fibrillation are present then treatment with antiarrhythmics should be continued for a longer period.

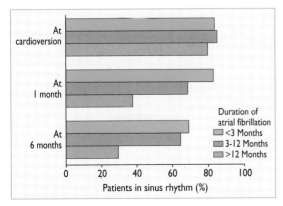

Patients in sinus rhythm at time of cardioversion and at one month and six months of follow up according to duration of atrial fibrillation.

Prognosis after cardioversion

A long previous duration of arrhythmia, previous episodes of atrial fibrillation, and age >50 years predict unsuccessful maintenance of sinus rhythm and reversion of atrial fibrillation. In addition, the presence of coronary artery disease, hypertension, and other organic disease—such as mitral valve disease, aortic stenosis, and cardiomyopathy—are detrimental to maintaining normal sinus rhythm.

Recent studies suggest that left atrial size does not influence the outcome after cardioversion but that the duration of atrial fibrillation is the most important predictor for outcome. Even with a dilated left atrium, long term sinus rhythm (about 80% at 12 months) is possible with the use of antiarrhythmic drugs.

Cardioversion of atrial fibrillation

Summary

- Cardioversion to sinus rhythm should be considered for all suitable patients in atrial fibrillation
- In the short term both pharmacological and electrical cardioversion restore sinus rhythm
- Prophylactic treatment with antiarrhythmic drugs is advisable after cardioversion in high risk patients in view of the high relapse rate
- Anticoagulants should be started before non-emergency cardioversion—ideally two to three weeks before—and continued for at least four weeks after cardioversion in patients with atrial fibrillation of >48 hours' duration

The duration of the arrhythmia seems to be the most important factor influencing prognosis after cardioversion. Twice as many patients who have had atrial fibrillation for less than three months remain in sinus rhythm as patients who have had atrial fibrillation for more than 12 months.

Key references

ACP/ACC/AHA Task Force Statement. Clinical competence in elective direct current (DC) cardioversion. *J Am Coll Cardiol* 1993;**22**:336–9

Clark A, Cotter L. Practical procedures—DC cardioversion. *Br J Hosp Med* 1991;**46**:114–5.

Laupacis A, Albers GW, Dunn JE, Dunn MI, Feinberg W, Jacobson AK. Antithrombotic therapy in atrial fibrillation. *Chest* 1995;**108**(suppl):352–9S

Lip GYH. Cardioversion of atrial fibrillation. *Postgrad Med J* 1995;**71**:457–65.

A more comprehensive version of this chapter can be found in Lip GYH, *Postgrad Med J* 1995;71:457–65.

The source of the data in the box of recommendations for anticoagulation before and after cardioversion is Laupacis A *et al*, *Chest* 1995;108(suppl):352–9S. The histogram was adapted from Dittrich *et al*, *Am J Cardiol* 1989;63:193-7.

8 ATRIAL FIBRILLATION IN GENERAL AND HOSPITAL PRACTICE

Gregory Y H Lip, D Gareth Beevers, John R Coope

General practice

Role of general practitioner

- To identify patients with new onset atrial fibrillation
- To assess thromboembolic risk and to start early treatment with antithrombotic drugs—warfarin will be needed for most patients, while aspirin may be suitable for patients aged <65 years with no cardiac risk factors or structural heart disease
- To help to monitor treatment with anticoagulants
- To refer appropriate patients to a cardiologist for further assessment (including echocardiography) and consideration of cardioversion
- To be aware of potential drug interactions and toxicity with antiarrhythmic drugs and anticoagulants

---

Despite the considerable interests in atrial fibrillation in epidemiological and hospital studies, little information exists on the prevalence and management of atrial fibrillation in general practice.

In a recent audit of a general practice list of about 10 000 patients, we found 67 patients who were currently in atrial fibrillation or who were known to have had past episodes of the arrhythmia.

A general practitioner typically has 10–15 patients with atrial fibrillation on his or her list

---

This prevalence increased with age, rising from 1·5% in people in their 60s to 8% in those aged over 90. A third of the 67 patients had paroxysmal atrial fibrillation. Only two thirds were currently receiving anticoagulant treatment, and an echocardiogram had been obtained in only a third. Of the 30 patients under 75 years, 10 had mitral valve disease, while only one patient aged over 75 had mitral valve disease.

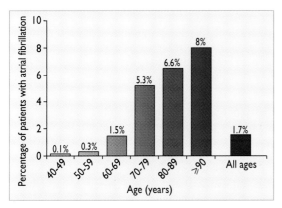

Prevalence of atrial fibrillation by age in a general practice population.

From the stroke prevention in atrial fibrillation study, major clinical risk factors for stroke and thromboembolism were congestive heart failure, hypertension, and previous thromboembolism. We found that at least one of these risk factors was present in three quarters of patients seen in general practice with atrial fibrillation (and in 84% of those aged over 75).

The general population is aging—that is, the proportion of elderly people is increasing—and by the year 2000 the proportion of people over 70 in Britain will constitute 20–25% of the total population. Atrial fibrillation will therefore be an increasingly common cause of stroke, thromboembolism, and heart failure, emphasising that atrial fibrillation is an important public health problem. Many patients will also be taking antiarrhythmic drugs and anticoagulants.

When to refer patients with atrial fibrillation to a cardiologist

Age <30
Atrial fibrillation resistant to "usual" drugs for rate control
Patient suitable for cardioversion
Further assessment needed—for example, valvar heart disease
Patient with moderate to severe heart failure
Patient with resistant heart failure
Frequent attacks of paroxysmal atrial fibrillation
Syncopal attacks due to atrial fibrillation

As many elderly patients have other medical conditions, the problem of side effects and drug interactions will become increasingly common. For example, hypokalaemia secondary to the use of high doses of loop diuretics may result in dangerous arrhythmias in patients taking digoxin. The use of antiarrhythmics such as amiodarone may result in drug interactions with warfarin and digoxin with consequent toxicity.

Such possibilities emphasise the need for concurrent treatments to be fully recorded and for a high index of suspicion for drug interactions. Non-compliance by patients because of inadequate understanding or supervision may also be dangerous. Careful monitoring of requests for repeat prescriptions is therefore essential.

Drugs that may interact with oral anticoagulants

Gastrointestinal tract
Potentiating drugs—Antacids (magnesium salts); cimetidine; liquid paraffin and other laxatives
Antagonistic drugs—Cholestyramine; colestipol

Cardiovascular system
Potentiating drugs—Amiodarone; clofibrate; dextrothyroxine; diazoxide; dipyridamole; ethacrynic acid; quinidine; sulphinpyrazone
Antagonistic drugs—Cholestyramine; colestipol; spironolactone

Respiratory system
Antagonistic drugs—Antihistamines

Central nervous system
Potentiating drugs—Chloral hydrate and related compounds; chlorpromazine; dextropropoxyphene; dichloralphenazone (initial); diflunisal; mefenamic acid; monoamine oxidase inhibitors; triclofos sodium; tricyclic antidepressants
Antagonistic drugs—Barbiturates; carbamazepine; dichloralphenazone—late; haloperidol; phenytoin; primidone

Infections
Potentiating drugs—Aminoglycosides; ampicillin (oral); cephalosporins; chloramphenicol; co-trimoxazole; cycloscerine; erythromycin; isoniazid; ketoconazole; metronidazole; miconazole; nalidixic acid; penicillin G (large doses)—intravenous; quinine salts; streptotriad; sulphonamides (long acting); tetracycline
Antagonistic drugs—Griseofulvin; rifampicin

Endocrine system
Potentiating drugs—Anabolic steroids; chlorpropamide; corticosteroids; danazol; glucagon; metoclopramide; propylthiouracil; sulphonyl urea; thyroxine; tolbutamide
Antagonistic drugs—Oral contraceptives

Malignant disease and immunosuppression
Potentiating drugs—Cyclophosphamide; mercaptopurine; methotrexate; immunosuppressant drugs; tamoxifen

Musculoskeletal and joint disease
Potentiating drugs—Allopurinol; aspirin and the salicylates; azapropazone; diflunisal; fenclofenac; fenoprofen; fluefenamic acid; flubiprofen; indomethacin; ketoprofen; mefenamic acid; naproxen; paracetamol (high daily doses with dextropropoxyphene (distalgesic/coproxamol)); piroxicam; sulindac; sulphinpyrazone

Nutrition and blood
Potentiating drugs—Alcohol (dose dependent potentiator)
Antagonistic drugs—Vitamin K; alcohol

Ear, nose and oesophagus
Antagonistic drugs—Antihistamines; phenazone

Skin
Antagonistic drugs—Antihistamines

Alcoholism
Potentiating drugs—Disulfiram (antabuse)

Who to screen for atrial fibrillation in general practice

Patients complaining of palpitations or syncope
Patients with stroke or transient ischaemic attacks
Patients with heart failure
Patients taking diuretics regularly or digoxin
Patients with thyroid disease

The increasing prevalence of atrial fibrillation will result in more patients taking anticoagulant drugs. A high proportion of patients in general practice have risk factors for thromboembolism, which necessitate long term treatment with anticoagulants. This presents two problems: inconvenience and safety. Patients taking warfarin need regular monitoring of anticoagulation intensity and adjustment of dosage. Although this is often done at specialist anticoagulation clinics either in hospitals or in the community, this task is now increasingly being undertaken by some general practitioners. Many general practitioners, however, may be reluctant to take on this responsibility.

Increasing numbers of patients needing warfarin would cause considerable strain on the current provision of anticoagulation monitoring services, and new initiatives to provide anticoagulation in the community are urgently needed. Frail elderly people should not have to attend hospital clinics, which may be some distance from their homes. The safety considerations are related to the risk of haemorrhage and of drug interactions.

With the potentially increasing importance of atrial fibrillation as a cause of mortality or morbidity, the question arises of whether screening programmes would be cost effective? All general practitioners should at least have easy access to a reliable electrocardiogram machine to confirm atrial fibrillation; electrocardiography is easy to perform, although careful placement of the leads and interpretation is needed. Some difficulties, however, may arise in distinguishing atrial fibrillation from other supraventricular arrhythmias and in identifying pre-excitation syndromes.

Open access to general practitioners for echocardiography in local hospitals for patients with heart failure has been tried successfully in some centres, and there is a good case for extending this facility to the management of atrial fibrillation.

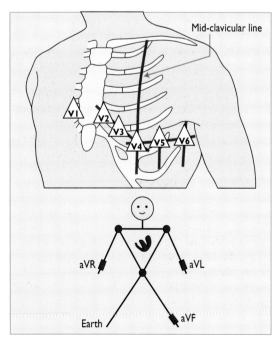

Standard positions for chest leads (top) and limb leads (bottom) for electrocardiography.

Atrial fibrillation in general practice—important considerations

Atrial fibrillation (continuous or intermittent) is an important cause of stroke in patients aged over 75

Most of these patients have other risk factors for strokes, including a history of hypertension, congestive heart failure, or previous thromboembolism

Thyroid disease should be excluded

Echocardiography may be valuable in these patients

Unless contraindicated, treatment with anticoagulants or prophylactic aspirin should be started

Vigilance is necessary for side effects or drug interactions

The adequate treatment of atrial fibrillation, as of other chronic diseases, needs an effective channel of communication between hospital and general practice. Decisions on the advantages and disadvantages of treatment with anticoagulants need to be made jointly by the physician, the general practitioner, and the individual patient. A realistic assessment should be made of the burden placed on older patients by medical intervention. Some may prefer to be left alone, and providing that they understand the risks and benefits of treatment, this wish, should of course, be respected.

Hospital practice

Cost (£) of cardiological investigations in patients with atrial fibrillation

Electrocardiogram	£10–24
Trace with cardiomemo machine	£33
Trace with 24 hour Holter monitor	£60
Echocardiogram (two dimensional and M mode only)	£72
Echocardiogram (with Doppler)	£147

Costs provided by cardiology department, City Hospital, Birmingham

Variation in treatment

- The quality of investigation and treatment of atrial fibrillation by non-specialist physicians varies
- A study in Britain of consultant physicians found that cardiologists did more detailed investigations than non-cardiologists
- Cardiologists were also more likely to use antiarrhythmic and antithrombotic treatment

As with general practice, the future increasing prevalence of atrial fibrillation will mean there will be more patients at increased risk of stroke and heart failure needing hospital care. In a Scottish hospital based study atrial fibrillation was present in 6·3% of emergency medical admissions. In our survey of admissions to a city centre district hospital in Birmingham covering a multiethnic population, atrial fibrillation was present in 3·3% of emergency admissions, with a lower proportion among black (Afro-Caribbean), and Asian people. In both surveys this arrhythmia was associated with a pronounced morbidity and mortality from heart failure, stroke, and syncope. However, in a local study of patients with atrial fibrillation in two west Birmingham general practices, only a third of patients ever presented to hospital, suggesting hospital based surveys may misrepresent the true prevalence and clinical features of atrial fibrillation in the community.

Atrial fibrillation has important implications for the provision of investigations, such as echocardiography. Most cardiologists use this investigation for their patients with atrial fibrillation. In patients presenting with syncope, 24 hour Holter monitoring is advisable. Syncope is common in patients with atrial fibrillation, and the question therefore arises whether we can afford to investigate all patients with atrial fibrillation with so many detailed and expensive procedures.

Implications for more anticoagulation clinics

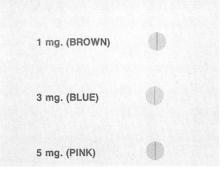

1 mg. (BROWN)

3 mg. (BLUE)

5 mg. (PINK)

Warfarin tablets available in Britain.

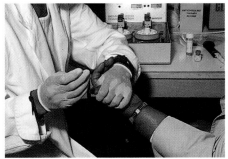

Taking a blood sample in an anticoagulation clinic.

Patients taking warfarin as thromboprophylaxis need to attend anticoagulation clinics regularly so that the international normalised ratio can be monitored. Warfarin has potentially serious haemorrhagic side effects, particularly in elderly people, in whom peptic ulcers are common. Furthermore, many drugs have potentially serious drug interactions with warfarin. Cimetidine, for example, may inhibit the metabolism of warfarin, resulting in overanticoagulation. People taking warfarin would also need well designed literature, written in non-technical language, about what to do in the event of unusual symptoms or signs of bleeding. If such patients rely on ambulances this adds to the overall costs of treating such patients. Our hospital runs domiciliary anticoagulation checks, which minimise this expense.

Recent studies suggest that outpatient anticoagulation clinics may be less than satisfactory, with fewer than 50% of the results falling within the therapeutic range and nearly one third of patients being classed as "poorly controlled." This may be due to the high workload and inadequate time available to communicate with patients. Patients may also have to travel a long way to the nearest clinic and so may not keep all their appointments.

Atrial fibrillation in general and hospital practice

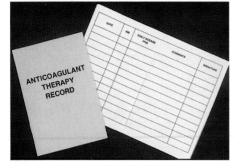

Booklet for recording anticoagulant treatment.

One solution may be more monitoring of anticoagulation treatment by general practitioners. A recent report suggests that the degree of anticoagulation control among patients in the care of general practitioners was better than that achieved by hospitals. If the benefits of anticoagulation treatment are to be extended to more patients with atrial fibrillation, particularly to older patients at higher risk, more attention will have to be given to the degree of control achieved. Only if this approaches that achieved in the large clinical trials will there be the substantial reduction of stroke reported in these trials.

The future

The future management of patients with artrial fibrillation will need to address two important considerations. Firstly, new developments in thromboprophylaxis are needed so that patients with atrial fibrillation are inconvenienced as little as possible and receive prophylaxis with maximal efficacy in preventing strokes and thromboembolism. Large scale randomised studies exploring the use of very low intensity warfarin and aspirin and combinations of these are currently in progress.

Secondly, the ability to identify patients with atrial fibrillation who are at high risk of thromboembolic complications would be an important advance. Although clinical risk factors for stroke have been identified for patients with atrial fibrillation, transthoracic echocardiography may further refine risk stratification. Recently, transoesophageal echocardiography has been similarly used—for example, in the risk stratification of such patients before cardioversion. Patients with atrial fibrillation have also been found to have a hypercoagulable or prothrombotic state, with abnormalities of indices of thrombogenesis. Clearly, further study of ways to stratify the risks of patients with atrial fibrillation is needed.

The source of the data in the histogram is unpublished (J R Coope). The data in the box on drugs that react with oral anticoagulants are adapted from British Society of Haematology, *J Clin Pathol* 1990;**43**:177-83.

Key references

British Society of Haematology. Guidelines on oral anticoagulation. *J Clin Pathol* 1990;**43**:177–83

Sudlow CM, Rodgers H, Kenny RA, Thomson RG, Sweeney KG, Pereira Gray DJ, *et al*. Service provision and use of anticoagulants in atrial fibrillation. *BMJ* 1995;**311**:558–60

Lip GYH, Zarifis J, Watson RDS, Beevers DG. Physician variation in the management of patients with atrial fibrillation. *Heart* 1996;**75**:200–5.

Pell JP, McIver B, Malone DNS, Alcock J. Comparison of anticoagulant control among patients attending general practice and a hospital anticoagulant clinic. *Br J Gen Pract* 1993;**43**:152–4.

Sweeney KG, Gray DP, Steele R, Evans P. Use of warfarin in non-rheumatic atrial fibrillation: a commentary from general practice. *Br J Gen Pract* 1995;**45**:153–8

Zarifis J, Beevers DG, Lip GYH. Acute admissions with atrial fibrillation in a British multiracial hospital population. *Br J Clin Pract* 1996 (in press).

INDEX

Abbreviations: AF, atrial fibrillation; CV, cerebrovascular

Index